Hypnobirthing

Judith Flood

Hypnobirthing

Judith Flood

Thank you to my husband (and birthing partner) Chris and my four beautiful boys.

An Association of Hypnobirthing Midwives Book
www.ahbm.co.uk

Created and produced by Judith Flood First published in Great Britain in 2012

Contents

Foreword

This text is intended as a guide and accompaniment to a Hypnobirthing Course led by a Hypnobirthing Midwife trained by the Association of Hypnobirthing Midwives.

Some women will birth easily and gently without learning about hypnobirthing or attending a Hypnobirthing Course. Others will need to spend time in preparation and contemplation, learning and practising techniques that will benefit themselves, their birthing partners and their babies during birth.

In the modern world we receive many negative messages about birth and, therefore for most women and their birthing partners it is imperative that they learn ways to counter these messages and to build their trust and confidence in their ability to birth.

The principles, ideas and philosophy of hypnobirthing are simple and straightforward and this text hopes to reflect that simplicity. Care has been taken to avoid information overload and to keep the ideas concise and the techniques suggested straightforward and easy.

If you are reading this and are unable to attend a course along side, it is highly recommended that you listen to a Hypnobirthing CD or MP3 track as well. Practice is key and daily practising is recommended for both the hypnobirthing mum and her birthing partner.

Notes

*The pregnant woman who is using hypnobirthing to prepare for her birth will be referred to as the 'hypnobirthing mum'.

*The 'birthing woman' or BW refers to a pregnant woman whose body is moving through the process of birth.

*The term 'birthing partner' or BP does not assume gender or the relationship to the birthing woman. It assumes a person who is with the birthing woman during her birthing as an advocate and supporter. It does not refer to someone who simply witnesses the birth as a bystander and the word 'partner' is deliberate as it suggests a shared experience and working toward a common goal.

*To protect confidentiality I have changed the names of all those mentioned in birth stories including work colleagues.

*The term 'hypnobirthing couple' refers to the birthing woman and her birthing partner. Is it assumed that in most cases the couple attends a hypnobirthing course together.

The Language of Hypnobirthing

In order to avoid the negative language all too often associated with childbirth hypnobirthing uses alternative words to the mainstream terminology. Listed below are examples of these;

**Surge* instead of contraction

**Birthing* instead of labour

**Early phase of birthing* instead of early labour or latent phase, a fuller description of the early phase is given in Chapter Twenty Three

**Active phase of birthing* instead of first stage of labour i.e. the part from about 4cm dilated up to fully dilated, see Chapter Twenty Four

**Birth* or *birthing phase* instead of the second stage of labour i.e. the actual birth itself when the baby is born.

Introduction

I will always remember the first 'Hypnobirthing' woman I ever met. I had arrived ten minutes late on the Birth Centre for a late shift because my young son, who was then just one year old, was unwell and we had both found the idea of me leaving him to go to work quite difficult.

So I had arrived at work somewhat distracted and somewhat hassled. I am normally almost compulsive about punctuality and being 10 minutes late bothered me. Katy, the midwife in charge that day, wasn't hassled or bothered in the slightest. It was unusually quiet on the Maternity Unit and so it gave everyone a very rare opportunity to take things a little slower for once. I remember I was the only midwife arriving for a late shift so, after the usual pleasantries, Katy leaned back in her chair and surveyed the relatively clear whiteboard which listed all the women who had been admitted to the birth centre.

'OK Judith, let's see...go and see the woman in room fifteen, she thinks she's in labour but she's not...you'll need to send her home.' she said with an apologetic smile.

My heart sank as I walked down the corridor to room fifteen. Telling a women she is not in the active stage of her birthing when she thinks she is and then sending her home is possibly one of my least favourite parts of being a midwife. There is evidence to suggest that a woman's birth will progress more smoothly if she stays at home as long as possible in earlier part of her birthing (Bailit et al 2005, Klein et al 2004, Homes et al 2001). Other research, however, has shown that some women might perceive that being told to stay at home by a midwife is more in the professional's best interests than hers (Nolan, Smith 2010).

In my experience this would be the typical course of events;

A woman is having her first baby - let's call her Mable. One afternoon she starts to feel strange tightening sensations in her bump, after three or four of these tightenings she notices they are painful. She stops for a moment. Oh my god, this is it, labour! Mable is scared of what lies ahead, she's not too sure what to expect, she is stressed and unprepared. So in an attempt to get a grip and some support she makes a semi-hysterical phone call demanding that her partner (let's call him Jim) return home from work immediately. Jim now is also in a panic and with a huge rush of adrenaline cycles madly home. Meanwhile, Mable, who is a bit excited but mainly scared decides to telephone her Mum, her Aunty, her friends and her neighbours to let them all know the baby is on it's way, hey she might even put a post on Facebook!

Now let's move on to three days later. Mable is still at home, still feeling lots of painful tightenings but still has not had her baby. She has made several calls to the midwives at the hospital asking if she can go there for some help, after all these painful tightenings are still coming, there's lots of pain and tightness and pressure. Every time she calls though she gets the same reply, 'It's too early to come in...you need to wait until things get stronger.' For three days now Mable's tense, fearful body has been braced against the onslaught of contractions. She's exhausted, dehydrated, has lost her appetite and now she has a new fear to add to the ones already flying around her head. The fear that her body just can't do this thing, that it's not able to get the baby out (in fact she had suspected this all along). This fear is compounded by the dozens of phone calls and texts she's now getting from friends and family asking, neigh demanding, to know where the baby is?! Finally, Mable feels under so much pressure that she decides to just turn up at the hospital, maybe then the midwives will see that she's not coping or realise that it's not that early because surely by now something should be happening. When Mable and Jim arrive at hospital they are already in a pretty bad place when they meet me! And of course I've seen this all before, hundreds of times - women and their birthing partners turning up on labour ward desperately wishing, hoping and almost willing themselves into the active phase of birth. And the message I give to Mable? Well it's usually that she's wrong, that she doesn't know her own body and what's more that it's all going to get much worse AND there's nothing anyone can do AND we can't accommodate you here so go home! Now, I like to think that myself and other midwives don't put it quite like that, but the reality is that there can be little support from birthing professionals for women who are not coping in the early phase of their birth . The answer to this therefore lies in preparation and understanding for women and their partners for this time - but I will come to that later.

So back to the woman in room fifteen who I now knew to be called Jenny. As I entered the room my heart sank even further. Jenny was sitting on a birthing ball, gently bouncing up and down and looking at the sunlit view out of the window, as soon as she saw me she turned, gave me a big smile and a cheery hello! My immediate assessment was that Jenny certainly was not in in the active phase of her birthing and I just hoped she wouldn't mind going home too much!

As it was a quiet day I had the luxury of taking my time with Jenny and hoped that at least she wouldn't feel rushed out. So we began to chat. I always like to meet and assess women this way, rather than with a whole list of questions. I prefer us to spend some time getting to know each other. Pregnant women almost without exception like to talk about their pregnancy, so it's easy to get a history just by 'having a chat' and it makes the whole thing seem so much less clinical and helps to build trust and rapport. Early on in our conversation Jenny asked if she could put on a 'hypnosis for childbirth CD' as she had had some hypnotherapy for her birth. I replied in the affirmative but didn't ask anymore as I didn't want to appear ignorant of the subject.

I was, however, very ignorant of the subject. I had a vague recollection of reading somewhere about hypnosis for birth whilst studying as a student midwife but my only experience of hypnosis up until that point was whilst I was a student nurse (a long, long time ago, in a student bar far, far away...). I recall watching a middle aged man in a bow tie enticing students up onto the stage to be hypnotised into thinking an onion was an apple or to forget the number 3! I thought it must be mind control or some kind of magic trick.

So once again back to Jenny in room fifteen! She was particularly calm and smiley I thought. Too calm and smiley to possibly to be in the active phase of her birth. Also every time she had a surge she would put her hand on the top of her bump and say 'Ooh there's one now' and continue to chat. Now I was *really* sure she wasn't far along in her birthing. I had been a midwife for nearly five years, had seen many births and I was very sure that a surge had to completely stop someone in their tracks to be strong enough. If Jenny could talk through her surges they simply weren't strong enough. So with a deep breath and a weak smile I said, 'Jenny, you're doing really well and I can see things are beginning to happen, but it's still early days and I think you need to go home for now. I'm sure the contractions will get much stronger and hopefully that will happen soon but if you want, before you leave, I can do an internal (vaginal examination) to give you some idea if the neck of the womb has started to open at all. It's up to you.'

I was thankful Jenny opted for the vaginal examination as the neck of her womb was six centimetres dilated and she was clearly well into the active phase of her birthing.. She went on to birth her baby around six hours later, very calmly and still smiling!

Of course I was hugely relieved that Jenny had opted for the internal and I that I didn't send her home but I was also fascinated by the calmness and power of her birth.

Chapter One

Jenny's birth was unusual. I had witnessed quick and easy births before but not often and rarely with first time mothers. I had witnessed a handful of births where women seemed to just be able to let go and 'give birth' so although I knew Jenny's peaceful, easy birth was unusual it wasn't unheard of.

A few weeks after witnessing Jenny's hypnobirth I arrived at the Birth Centre for an early shift and was asked to be with a woman called Natalie who had arrived there, with her birthing partner, about an hour earlier. As I entered the room I noticed Natalie was listening to the same CD that Jenny had played during her birth, I remember thinking it was quite a coincidence. Natalie's birth was very different to Jenny's of course, as all births are completely unique, but it had the same air of calmness and peace about it. Just before I arrived Natalie had agreed for the midwife on the night shift to carry out a vaginal examination which had shown that the neck of the womb was 4cm dilated. As I met her it was obvious her body was actively birthing with long, powerful surges.

Throughout my time with Natalie I sat and silently observed her with increasing wonder, she appeared to be really concentrating most of the time and her breathing was very slow and very deep. Occasionally she would come out of her reverie to communicate with either myself or her partner but soon, with a deep breath, she would drift off again. For much of the time she walked round and round the room slowly and with purpose. She would stop during a surge to breathe and sway, the whole thing was very hypnotic. The hypnobirthing CD was on in the background, it played very quietly and was only just audible and from time to time Natalie's partner read a hypnobirthing script (see Chapter 12) to her again very quietly.

As we approached midday Natalie agreed to another vaginal examination and this time the cervix was 9cm dilated so she continued for a while in the same vein, walking, breathing and swaying. I was simply a bystander watching in awe. Around an hour later Natalie told me that she had some strong urges to push. I remember this so clearly because I was almost amused as she looked at me, smiled and said, very calmly 'oh I think I need to push now'. She then proceeded to kneel down on the mat on the floor and for the next twenty minutes or so with deep, long breaths her baby very gently and yet with great efficiency began to slide into the outside world. As more and more of the baby appeared I looked on incredulously as Natalie leaned forwards slightly, took her own baby and lifted the newborn straight up to her chest. The total confidence of this act was incredible and would have been a very confident way to birth even for a woman who had birthed before, but this was Natalie's first baby, it was truly amazing.

I spent a couple of hours with Natalie after the birth and once again I was full of wonder, this time at how she viewed and talked about her experience of birth. I distinctly remember her saying, 'That was fantastic, I'd do it again tomorrow!' Something I had never, up to that point, heard a woman say straight after birthing. Incidentally since then, it is something I have only ever heard women say after hypnobirthing.

Over the next few months I witnessed a number of Hypnobirths. Each birth would be different from the last and each couple would use the hypnobirthing techniques differently. They did, however, all had a hallmark of calmness, control and confidence. Witnessing these births was inspiring and I wanted to know more. I needed to understand how it worked. From what I had seen so far it was easy to see how having mechanisms to help you and your birthing partner to relax could be helpful. I could see how breathing well and feeling relaxed could enhance your experience, but what fascinated me was that, it seemed to me, that women birthing their first babies using hypnobirthing seemed to have quicker births. What I have come to call 'efficient' births. Not quick and furious births like some women describe where the baby is born so quickly that they cannot cope mentally or physically but also not the long, drawn out birthings that are sadly so commonplace. It wasn't uncommon for hypnobirthing women to birth their first baby in 4, 6 or 8 hours. The birthing body doing it's job quickly and easily. Witnessing this really motivated me to find out more - how could a deep breath and having the ability to stay calm and positive have an effect on the whole process of birth - how could that be?

A few months after watching Jenny and Natalie and their phenomenal hypnobirths I once again had the privilege of seeing another beautiful and inspiring birth. This time I was on a night shift and I sat and watched Andrea as she serenely floated around in the birthing pool, birthing her first baby. Andrea had arrived in hospital at 8cm dilated, in itself quite an achievement! For most of her birthing she appeared very sleep like and utterly serene. Every so often she would open her eyes and say 'wow that was a strong one' and then close her eyes and drift off again. Her partner sat very close to her and occasionally reminded her to breathe deeply by very gently whispering in her ear. The pool room was dim and peaceful and much of the time the only sound was the gentle splashing of the water as Andrea rocked and swayed with her surges. A newly qualified midwife sat quietly by my side, this was her first hypnobirth and we sat together in quiet reverence to the inspiring events unfolding in the room. Andrea didn't need or want anything and our job was simply to watch and wait. After a while the new midwife leaned over to me, 'How do we know when she's having a contraction?' she whispered. I smiled and whispered back, 'We don't!'. It was impossible to tell when Andrea's surges began or ended as she appeared so sleep like most of the time. We had to trust Andrea's ability to birth just as much as she trusted herself.

As dawn broke Andrea birthed her baby into the water with stunning power. Her birthing body worked hard but again there was calmness, focus and total control. As Andrea's little boy swam up and out of the water he blinked a little in the dim light of the room and began to breathe without crying or complaining. Andrea held him close, kissed him and put him to her breast, he fed easily and quietly. It was a perfect birth.

As I arrived home that morning I didn't think about sleep. I sat down at the computer and typed 'Hypnosis for Childbirth' into google.

I needed to know more.

Chapter Two

After noticing how different birth could be for women using hypnobirthing I became more and more curious and began to read as much as I could on the subject. What I read made perfect sense. The ideas certainly weren't new either, it was more a renaissance, a re-birth of birth, you might say.

Who started Hypnobirthing?

It's not clear who first used the term 'Hypnobirthing' but the idea of using hypnosis for birth goes back many years.

James Braid, a Scottish surgeon who is often referred to as the founder of hypnotherapy describes using hypnotism to induce a woman's birth as early as 1853 (Robertson, 2009).

The idea of preparation and contemplation for birth is evident in many cultures. The American Indigenous Indians, for example, traditionally spent much time and care in preparation for childbirth. Adrien Van der don, a Dutch Colonialist, described a woman's preparation for childbirth among the Mohawk and Mahican Indians in the 17th Century, he wrote that pregnant women would;

'...depart alone to a secluded place near a brook, or stream of water . . . and prepare a shelter for themselves with mats and coverings, where, provided with provisions necessary for them, they await their delivery without the company or aid of any person. . . . They rarely are sick from child-birth [and] suffer no inconveniences from the same.'

This suggests mental and physical preparation for the event that lay ahead.

Even within modern culture there is a wide acknowledgment of the importance of preparation for childbirth. Most parents to be will seek out some kind of information during pregnancy either in the form of antenatal classes, reading or even just talking to others who had already experienced birth. There is a wealth of comment and some research supporting the idea that knowledge is empowering for birthing women and that antenatal education is beneficial. (Spinelli et al, 2003).

Hypnotherapy has been seen for many years as a useful method of preparation for birth, acknowledging the intrinsic connection between the mind and the body for this act which is so physical and yet so psychological at the same time. Who first thought of the idea of putting these ideas into an antenatal programme and coining the term 'Hypnobirthing' is difficult to tell. Marie Mongan, an American Hypnotherapist claims it was her idea and her hypnobirthing book is probably the best selling hypnobirthing book on the market. Michelle Le Claire O'Neil, an American nurse, however, claims she thought of it first and that Marie Mongan simply marketed the ideas more vigorously and, therefore, became more well known. This dispute ended with a court ruling where a judge in New Hampshire in the United States ruled that Mongan could call her progamme 'HypnoBirthing - The Mongan Method' and O'Neill could call hers 'The Original Method' (Mongan was only allowed to trademark the word hypnobirthing with a capital B for birthing - for Judge's ruling via weblink see referencing). Mongan then attempted twice more in the United Kingdom and the European Union to register the word hypnobirthing as her own trademarked name but was turned down each time on the grounds that it is now 'common parlance' to put the word 'hypno' with 'birthing' in order to describe the use of hypnosis for birth. In Canada four similar applications by Mongan were abandoned presumably on the grounds that they were unlikely to be upheld. In short anyone is free to use the word hypnobirthing to describe the use of hypnosis for childbirth and in the United States the only term to be trademarked is the stylised form of the word hypnobirthing with a capital B for birthing.

The real credit for the ideas of hypnobirthing goes to Dr. Grantley Dick-Read. Often referred to as 'The Father of Natural Childbirth' and his book 'Childbirth without Fear', first published in 1942 has become a true classic. Dick-Read was born in 1890 and fought in the first world war. His work as an obstetrician in the Eastend of London in the 1920's and 30's was the basis for his inspiration. Watching women birthing, often in the slums of the Eastend he started to theorise about the connection between the fear and pain of childbirth as well as developing the idea that women's expectations of childbirth often play out in reality. That is, if a woman expects childbirth to be difficult and painful then it probably will be, but if they trust they are able to do it then they will. Grantly Dick-Read had many exciting and progressive ideas about childbirth and very much trusted a woman's ability to birth. His radical ideas were not popular among his peers at the time and at one point he was even expelled from his clinic by his fellow Obstetricians. Later in his life he became a founding member of the Natural Childbirth Association (now the National Childbirth Trust) and since that time his ideas have been embraced the world over.

Grantly Dick-Read was a man way ahead of his time and yet at the same time he was taking birth back to basics, to it's natural form. His hypothesis about the connection between fear of birth and the pain experienced form the corner stone of hypnobirthing and, therefore it is essential that anyone planning on using hypnobirthing for their birth must have a clear understanding of the link between the two (Chapter Three describes this connection in detail). This understanding will mean that the hypnobirthing woman and her birthing partner will see the true importance of calmness, confidence and trust for birth as well as the need for allowing the birth to remain undisturbed.

Chapter Three

The Fear Tension Pain Cycle

Grantly Dick-Read's theories about the connection between pain and fear for women during childbirth are sensible, logical and rational. Those ideas are based on the changes that take place within the body when the Fight or Flight response or reflex is triggered.

Picture this, you are walking home after a long, hard day at work, your exhausted, hungry and dehydrated. You can't decide whether you'll eat when you get home or just fall straight into bed. It's fairly late now and dark, so you decide to take a short cut across a small park near your house. The park is normally very busy during the day but now it is deserted and dimly lit. As you drag your weary body onwards you suddenly sense movement in the shadows. You feel a strange chill. What was it? A cat, a fox or a stranger lurking in the shadows? Then there is another sudden movement and this time you think you see the outline of a Shrek-like figure skulking in the bushes and you're sure they mean harm. So now you run, run like the wind, faster than you've run for years and you're out of that park in seconds. As you arrive at your front door less than a minute later you suddenly remember again how tired you are and you notice how hard your heart is beating but strangely you're not hungry now just very, very tired.

In this situation the Fight of Flight response and the hormone Adrenaline have served you well, potentially kept you from harm or even saved your life. How incredible, that despite being so very tired, your body was able to respond instantly and so powerfully when you really needed it to. So let's breakdown what was happening in this scenario; Firstly, as you sensed danger and became afraid, you triggered the Fight or Flight response in the mind and the body and your body released a whole load of adrenaline - *an adrenaline rush*. The term 'Fight of Flight' refers to the body's response to a threatened or survival situation. In short that response will mean we will either stay and 'Fight' for survival or to run away and take 'Flight' in order to survive.

So now the Adrenaline rushing round your bloodstream sends your body into immediate 'Alpha Mode' and helps you release energy you didn't even know you had. It has also enabled you to focus on the potential danger, the only thought in your head now being the threatening figure in the bushes. You no longer think about your hard day at work or how exhausted you are, your senses are heightened and all you think about is getting out of the park. Anyone observing you might notice your dilated pupils, making your vision much more acute. They might even notice your nostrils flaring and your breathing becoming more rapid as your airways dilate and your body increases the uptake of oxygen. The 'danger' centre in your brain jump starts your body and the response is instantaneous. At the same time the adrenal glands (which lie just above the kidneys) pump the adrenaline into your blood stream. This adrenaline then signals to the liver to release glucose for energy and to the heart to beat faster and more strongly and so the circulation quickly races round the muscles. To aid your Olympic style sprint through the park the Fight or Flight reflex will facilitate the release of Adenosine Tri-Phosphate (ATP) which will help you to tap into energy that your body stores especially for emergency situations, a bit like a high energy emergency battery. ATP will turbo charge your body in a flash but only for a for a very short time, just a few seconds in fact, but that will give you the spurt you need to get out of danger.

The benefits of the Fight or Flight response and adrenaline in such a scenario speak for themselves but it is important to remember that these benefits are short lived. Once away from the potential danger in the park the rush of adrenaline has stopped and the 'come down' will begin. Coming down from an adrenaline rush is exhausting and can often be associated with a low mood or even depression (http://www.clinical-depression.co.uk 2012) As you arrived at your front door you noticed that not only were you suddenly extremely exhausted, you no longer felt hungry either. One action of adrenaline is to divert blood towards the vital organs (mainly the heart, lungs and brain) so they serve you well for the Fight or Flight. The side effect of this, however, is that blood is diverted away from the rest of the body, so the stomach, for example, will have a decreased blood supply which will inhibit the appetite.

What, you may ask, has any of this got to do with childbirth? Well, if during birth a woman feels stressed or afraid she will trigger the Fight or Flight Response and adrenaline will be released into her blood stream. Although, as we have seen adrenaline can be a useful hormone, in the case of the birthing body it is downright unhelpful. One of the reasons for this is because adrenaline is known to suppress the release of the birthing hormones, which are mainly Oxytocin and Endorphins. When a birthing body has a good flow of Oxytocin and Endorphins it will work easily and efficiently. However, if these hormones are blocked by adrenaline the birthing body can try all it likes to birth but it simply won't have what it needs to do the job well.

Endorphins

Grantly Dick-Read in his book 'Childbirth without Fear' wrote about the importance of birthing women being allowed to remain undisturbed during childbirth and to be able to relax for the sake of the 'neuromusulcar harmony' of their birthing bodies. He also observed that for birthing women who were free of fear that something 'wonderful' happened within their bodies that would make their births easier. Many of his peers scoffed at such ideas and he was shunned by his profession at the time. In fact, it wasn't until some 15 years after his death (in 1959) that Endorphins were discovered and he was in fact proved to be correct.

Endorphins were first discovered in 1974 by two separate groups of scientists. The term endorphin is actually an abbreviation of 'endogenous morphine' meaning the 'morphine' produced naturally in the body. Studies have shown that endorphins can be up to 80 times more powerful than morphine in their effect on the body (Horace et al 1976) and that raised levels are often found in women during childbirth (Contos 1981). Classically endorphins are associated with being a hormone that is released as the body's own natural pain killer but pain isn't necessarily needed for their release. Excitement, sexual arousal, happiness, love and even spicy foods can all trigger their effusion.

Interestingly long distance runners and endurance athletes will often describe feelings of relaxation, euphoria and happiness as they push themselves to their physical limits. These feelings suggests endorphin release so it seems that pain is not the only requirement for their release.

If the Fight or Flight response and the subsequent rush of adrenaline is avoided then endorphins will serve the BW enabling her to feel calm, relaxed and comfortable, therefore, making birth easier.

Oxytocin

'Oxytocin is the hormone of love, and to give birth without releasing this complex cocktail of love chemicals disturbs the first contact between the mother and the baby..It is this hormone flood that enables a woman to fall in love with her newborn and forget the pain of birth." Michelle Odent 2006.

The word oxytocin comes from the Greek for 'quick birth' and is a hormone most associated with the contracting of the uterus during birth and the expulsion of the placenta. It is released during breastfeeding and is mainly responsible for the ejection of the milk from the breast. Oxytocin has also been shown to be released during orgasm, pair bonding and mothering behaviours and it is often referred to as the 'love hormone'(Carmichael,1987). Studies where subjects have received intranasal Oxytocin have shown recipients to be less fearful, more trusting, more generous and more empathetic. (Baumgartner 2008, Ditzen 2008)

During childbirth huge pulses of oxytocin surge around the birthing body. This will cause the womb to squeeze or contract which in turn opens the neck of the womb. Oxytocin will assist the womb to push down and birth the baby as well as the placenta and this same action will also help prevent bleeding.

So the benefits of oxytocin and endorphins to the birthing body are undeniable and the BW must allow these hormones to flow and not be inhibited by the unnecessary release of adrenaline.

Also worth noting is that there is some evidence to suggest that the use of Epidural Anesthesia may be responsible for lower levels of oxytocin in women during childbirth. This may be one explanation as to why some births will slow down or even stop where an epidural is in place (Rahm 2002).

From all this it would be reasonable to conclude that birth is a truly hormonal act. To allow the birthing body to work in perfect harmony the BW must be able to feel relaxed, secure and free of distraction or disruption. The techniques and principles of hypnobirthing allow this to be the case.

Fight or Flight and the Uterus

So far we can see that fear is detrimental not just on an emotional level but also because it can cause a hormonal imbalance during birthing which will be unhelpful to say the least. There is another action that adrenaline can have on the birthing body which is equally unhelpful. As mentioned previously, adrenaline causes the diversion of blood away from the body towards the heart, brain and lungs as part of the Fight or Flight reflex. The extra and immediate work necessary for the vital organs in a Fight or Flight situation means they need an instant increase in blood supply. Therefore, the circulation in other areas of the body will decrease in order for the blood to be sent to where it is needed the most. Remember the scenario described earlier, of being afraid whilst taking a short cut through the park? Remember I mentioned 'you feel a strange chill'? Feeling cold is often associated with feeling fearful and it's not unusual to use phrases such as 'my blood ran cold' or 'I went cold' to describe a reaction to being afraid. This experience is likely to be as a result of the peripheral circulation in the skin shutting down whilst the circulation in the vital organs and muscles, that are needed for the Fight or Flight, increase.

Leading on from this another part of the body where the circulation will decrease during the Fight or Flight response will be in the uterus or womb. In a survival or threatened situation a good blood supply to the uterus is not vital so the circulation or blood supply there will decrease as blood is diverted to where it's needed more. This is fine if the situation is a survival one but during childbirth this can only be unhelpful. The uterus like any other part of the human body needs a good blood supply to do it's job well. The blood passing through the tissues of the uterus will take with it the oxygen and nutrients necessary to give the uterus the energy it needs to do it's work. And let's not forget that the uterus does indeed have some work to do - to get a baby from the inside to outside takes work and energy and a blood supply will act as the fuel for the uterus to be able to do it well.

So what happens to a uterus deprived of a good circulation? The answer is that like any muscle with an inhibited blood supply it will go into spasm or seize. Any muscle that doesn't have what it needs to function properly (i.e. the hydration, electrolytes and oxygen carried in the blood supply) will cramp as each muscle fibre becomes involuntarily tense. Most of you reading this will have at some point experienced that sudden painful onset of a muscle cramp, you may have even been woken in the night with it. If you have you'll remember the tightness in the muscle as well as the sudden and intense pain often associated with it. Cramp occurs as a result of a temporary, impeded blood supply to the muscle and so that muscle cannot function properly until the circulation improves.

The uterus is no exception to this and will too become tense, go into spasm or seize if it's blood supply is affected. It will inevitably struggle to do it's job if it does not have the energy source (provided by the blood supply) it so needs.

Hormonal Harmony and Undisturbed Birth

It is reasonable to assume that adrenaline will work against a birthing body making the experience more difficult and more painful. It is also, therefore, reasonable to assume that a good supply of oxytocin and endorphins will make the experience of birth easier. Birth is a hormonal, instinctive event. Pregnant women may hear or read much advice about childbirth and many spend a good number of hours attending antenatal classes full of information about birth. However what they cannot learn in a class or from a book is actually *how* to give birth. They might learn practical tips on managing the process or ways to help the process along but they cannot learn to initiate the surges or open the cervix. They cannot do this because it is deeply, innately programmed into the female body. In other words, it does it all by itself.

When I was younger we owned a cat who had kittens. To birth her kittens she found the warmest, darkest, most peaceful spot in the flat. The spot she found was perfect for her, it was soft, comfortable and very safely tucked away. This spot, however, just happened to be a box of winter jumpers that I had stored underneath the bed. The only way we knew she was there was because she could hear her gently purring as she quietly birthed her kittens (purring in cats is thought to release endorphins, Foster 2011). As we peered under the bed to see what was happening it became obvious why she had chosen to birth right there. It was very difficult to see and had we tried (which we didn't) it would have been just as difficult to reach, making it peaceful and secure for her to birth her offspring. Although I wished she had found another place besides my winter wardrobe to give birth I was not tempted for a moment to move her. I knew that should she be disturbed the birth would be inhibited or even stop altogether as her and her kittens safety would be threatened as she would perceive that it wouldn't be safe to give birth. The Fight or Flight would protect her from harm by stopping or slowing down the birthing.

Transfer this principle to birthing women and it is clear that being able to feel relaxed, undisturbed and secure are completely essential to birth going well.

In her article 'Out of the Laboratory: Back to the Darkened Room', the late Tricia Anderson, (2002) brilliantly compares the instinctive nature of cats birthing in peaceful, secure and dark places to the bright, clinical labour ward that can too often make women feel vulnerable. She argues that maybe the need for intervention during birth is more as a result of women feeling disturbed, distracted, unsafe and overstimulated, she says,

'If we revisit the basic physiology of birth and accept that it is hormone-driven, it becomes obvious why childbirth does not work well in 'laboratory' (hospital labour ward) conditions. Very simply, we know that slow pulses of oxytocin are needed to make the muscles of the uterus contract. We know that powerful pain-relieving morphine-like endorphins are then released when the body enters periods of high stress that help a woman cope with the intensity of those contractions, taking her off into a withdrawn, dreamlike state. We know that there will be a lull between the first and second stages as oxytocin production decreases with the loss of pressure on the now fully dilated cervix. We know that as the fetus descends in the second

stage there is another huge surge of oxytocin created by the distension of the vaginal vault that causes expulsive contractions, and that again in the third stage another surge in oxytocin causes the empty uterus to contract and the placenta to sheer off. We know that at the moment of birth, mother and baby have extraordinarily high levels of oxytocin and endorphins. These are never repeated at any other time in their lives, making them alert, open and receptive to each other .'

Anderson argues that in order for the birthing hormones to be released and the birth to proceed naturally the BW must feel totally safe, secure and undisturbed. She suggests that for many women home birth is the answer, as most women will feel much more secure and less disturbed in their own familiar surroundings. The use of hypnosis and being practised at inducing the hypnotic or deeply relaxed state means that hypnobirthing women can 'switch off' from potential disturbance and distraction and go to that 'dreamlike' state anytime, anywhere. Also the confidence and trust that hypnobirthing gives women in their ability to birth brings with it security and control even if an environment that might not promote it.

Tricia Anderson's article is one of the most inspirational pieces I have ever read regarding undisturbed birth and in my opinion should be read by every pregnant woman as part of her preparation for birth. So too should every birth professional read it and consider if their practice allows birth to remain peaceful, secure and undisturbed.

Pain

So far we have established that fear will trigger the Fight of Flight reflex which cause a surge of adrenaline in the body. Adrenaline will not only suppress the release of the birthing hormones it will cause the womb to become tense as a result of an impeded blood supply. This cramping of the muscle fibres in the womb will inevitably be associated with pain.

Pain is an essential, vital and protective sense in the body. It is a reflex and a very useful one at that. The pain you might experience if you put your hand on a hotplate would cause you to very quickly remove your hand and, therefore prevent or minimize any damage to it. Innately in all of us is the instinctive idea that pain means there is danger, that something is wrong and something needs to change. So if the BW feels unbearable, unmanageable and overwhelming pain her brain will constantly be perceiving danger and she will feel threatened. This in itself can trigger the Fight or Flight, the very thing that needs to be avoided during birth. A further discussion about pain and childbirth can be found in Chapter Five.

Grantly Dick-Read described this cyclical connection between fear and pain as the Fear, Tension, Pain Cycle and the illustration on the next page shows the sequence of events that can occur if the Fight or Flight is triggered. It shows not only the connection between fear of childbirth and the pain experienced but also the detrimental effect adrenaline can have on the whole process of birth itself.

The good news is that hypnobirthing principles and techniques release fears, build confidence and avoid overstimulating the BW thus avoiding triggering the Fight of Flight.

The Fear, Tension, Pain Cycle

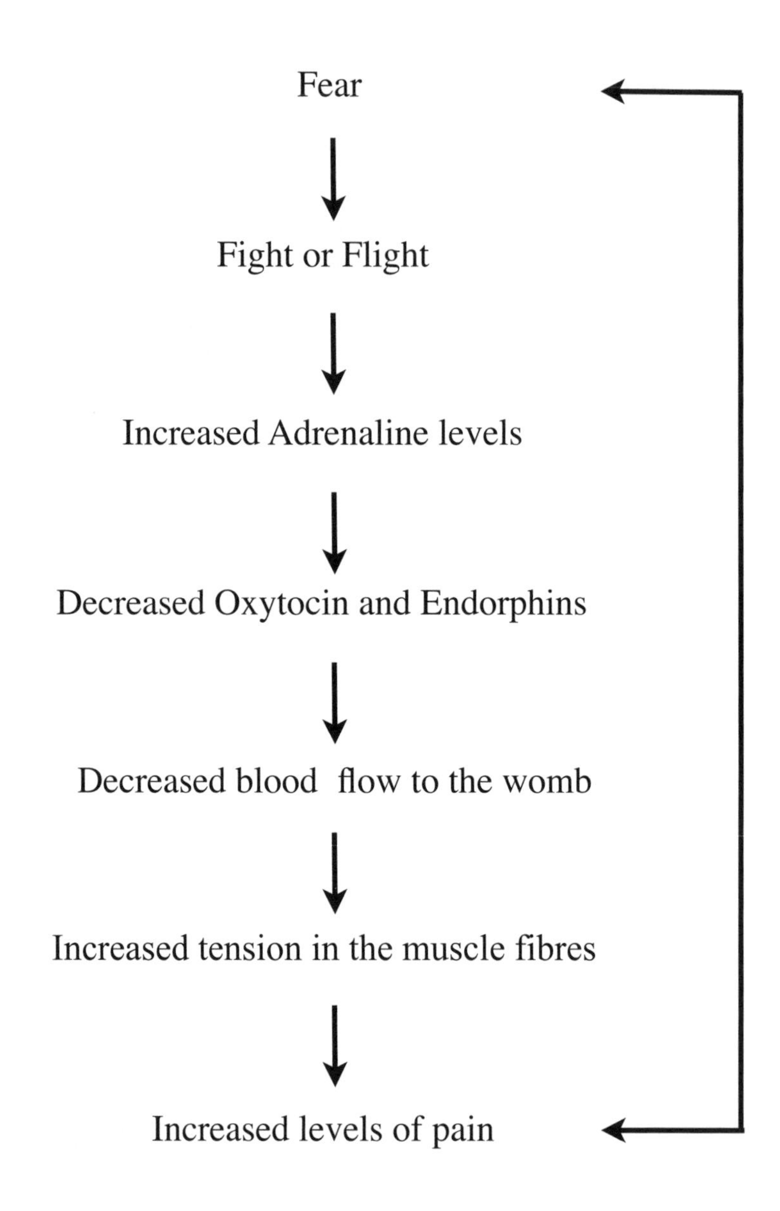

From the illustration on the previous page it's easy to see the connection between fear and pain during birth. Also what is patently clear is the effect that the Fight or Flight response can have on the whole process and physiology of birth.

A good few years ago I attended a birth which dramatically demonstrated the power of adrenaline on a woman's birthing body. I had been qualified for just a few months and although it was before I had even heard of hypnobirthing in retrospect I can now appreciate that this birth was so natural that it was a hypnobirth in nature if not in name. The couple were Tola and Aaron and Tola was inspiring to watch. She had a very long and lean body and I remember admiring the beauty with which all the muscles in her limbs were clearly defined. She marched and stomped her way around the room for the majority of the birth, stopping only for a surge during which she would sink into a semi-squat whilst breathing noisily and deeply. Her power and strength were undeniable. Around midday Tola expressed a strong urge to push and she felt she was ready to birth. Using a mat and a beanbag Tola adopted an all fours position on the floor and now with every surge her breathing, still long, deep and audible, changed to a long and purposeful blowing out. During this time I had become mesmerised by Tola's birthing and had not taken too much notice of Aaron as he seemed to have faded into the background. Aaron was a mild mannered, extremely thin man, who when I'd met him at the beginning of my shift, had greeted me with a big grin and sparkling eyes and seemed genuinely excited at the prospect of seeing his new baby soon. He had been working the night before as he was a security guard and had been called by Tola towards the end of his shift to say that her birthing was beginning. He told me with some pride that he hadn't slept in the last 24hrs and also that he hadn't left Tola's side since he had arrived home from work that morning. But as Tola's birthing had progressed he had moved further away from her both physically, sitting in the chair at the other side of the room, but also, it seemed, emotionally as his words of encouragement had become further and further apart. Non of this really mattered though as Tola was totally in her own world. She was very focused and when asked she replied that she didn't need or want anything. After a short time myself and Aaron witnessed that moment in any birth that is truly magical and never stops being so no matter how many births you might see. The top of the baby's head peeped out during a surge, the black curls of the baby's hair glistening in the light. At this precise moment, I'm not quite sure why, Aaron stood up quite suddenly and almost as suddenly fell to the floor and fainted. As he slumped to the floor, in a desperate, instinctive attempt to save or stop himself he managed to grab hold of the fetal heart monitor that was by his side (a real tank of a machine) and pulled that over too. And that wasn't all because on top of the monitor sat a jug full of water which also came splashing and crashing down with Aaron and the monitor. All this resulted in the most chaotic and dramatic scene anyone would *not* wish for during their birthing. The noise of the monitor crashing to the ground was tremendous and a litre of water on the floor suddenly felt like ten litres! My instinct was to ring the emergency bell, which in retrospect wasn't a good move because at least six midwives and doctors came crashing 'ER style' through the door, only adding to the disarray.

Among all the confusion I noticed that something quite incredible had happened to Tola. Her face had lost it's focused and purposeful look and she now looked understandably shocked and concerned. She was very concerned for Aaron, who by now had been guided into the nearest chair by one of the midwives and his head unceremoniously put between his knees. But, interestingly, the birthing and the surges had completely stopped. The sweet little head was still visible at the vulva and the baby's heartbeat remained perfectly normal as it had done so throughout the birth but Tola now had no urges to push and no surges either. The time from Aaron's involuntary lie down to everything being mopped and cleared up (by a crack team of midwives, who were very experienced in mopping up stuff of the floor) was around 20 minutes. In this time Tola's birthing completely stopped and then as things got (relatively) back to normal the surges started again, slowly at first but then once again they became strong and powerful and the birthing continued. Around 30 minutes later a gorgeously round baby was in his mother's arm, contented at his mother's breast.

Since being at Tola's birth I have been careful to explain to all birthing partners how important it is that they look after themselves during a birthing. Aaron hadn't had any sleep and out of pure concern and love he had not left Tola's side once. His stoicism had meant he hadn't eaten or drunk anything either. At the point at which he could see his baby arriving he stands up quickly and his poor tired, dehydrated body just can't cope, so he faints. Tola's body on the other hand has instantly triggered the Fight or Flight reflex as she senses potential danger and so her birthing body temporarily halts the birth as a protective measure.

As mankind has evolved the female body's ability to stop or slow down their birth in a dangerous or threatened situation would have been key. The pause in proceedings would enable her to move to a safe place to birth, away from predators or other dangers. This would have been essential to our survival and ultimately our evolution.

Once the calamity was over Tola's birthing body took over again and the birthing continued - no problem - how amazingly, beautifully clever!

More often, however, adrenaline will make a birthing long, difficult and painful. Too many birth stories talk about hours and hours of painful labour, of the cervix refusing to dilate or getting stuck, of babies sitting high up in the womb and struggling to descend into the pelvis. The question remains then that if the Fight or Flight and adrenaline are responsible for a birth that slows down or stops is the appropriate action to intervene with artificial and technological means such as syntocinon drips or forceps? Or would these births benefit more from encouraging and promoting the flow of oxytocin and endorphins by providing the BW with a peaceful and safe place to birth?

So it's easy to see that if a BW is to allow her birthing body to do the job it is perfectly well designed to do, she needs to eliminate fear, feel safe and free of distraction and fully trust in the whole process of birth and in her own body's ability to birth.

This means that preparation is key. Preparation on two levels. Firstly the preparation of understanding, knowing exactly how the birthing body works but also mental and emotional preparation, the two must go together.

Chapter Four

Knowledge is power

Many hours of Midwives' time are spent reassuring women that what is happening to them and their bodies during their birthing is perfectly normal and nothing to worry about. I was once with a woman called Asha during her birthing who, a few hours earlier, had lost the mucus plug that sits in the cervix during pregnancy. The mucus plug, often called a 'show', forms throughout pregnancy and provides a seal a which will protect the unborn baby from any bacteria that might find it's way towards the womb. Asha's mucus plug had come away early in her birthing and it happened to have a fair amount of blood mixed with it. To have some blood mixed in with a show is perfectly normal (as opposed to 'period type' bleeding without the presence of mucus which must always be checked out by a midwife) but Asha had seen blood and could only think this signaled a problem and she was terrified. I began to explain to Asha what the mucus plug was and that it had been in her cervix to protect her baby (how amazing is that!). Then I went on to tell her that the reason she had seen the plug in her pants was because the neck of the womb had (very cleverly!) thinned out and opened up to start the process of letting her baby out and in that process the plug had been released. Next I explained that nearly always the show brings some blood with it but that is a reassuring sign that the cervix was indeed changing.

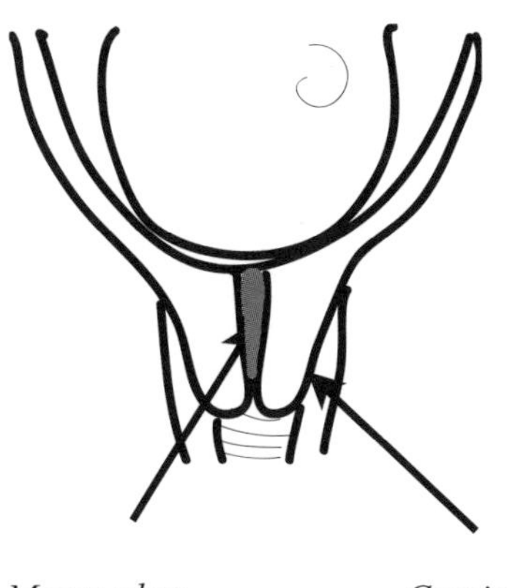

Unfortunately all this was too late for Asha, she was overwhelmed by fear and pain and I felt it was impossible for me to pierce the fearful mist that surrounded her. If only she could have embraced the whole idea of the show being a wonderful outward sign of amazing internal change. Understanding that her cervix was thinning and opening all by itself, that she didn't need to think about it or put any conscious effort into it - that her birthing body was on autopilot and knew exactly what it was doing. In this knowledge she would have been able to celebrate the mucus plug knowing that it brought her nearer to meeting her baby and be inspired at how phenomenal her birthing body was! Instead, her blind panic meant that she spent the whole time feeling very scared that she was bleeding and in fact expressed more than once that she was worried that she might die. She became stuck physically as well and seemed unable to get up off the bed. Surely enough, the birthing slowed and finally stalled altogether and ended in the inevitable trip to theatre.

The good news for birthing women is that it really does not have to be like this, it *is* possible for a woman to have such trust and confidence in her birthing body that she can celebrate and welcome each physical change that her body goes through. A hypnobirthing mum once said to me that she 'welcomed' each surge as she knew each one brought her nearer to meeting her baby and that she felt her body was so incredibly clever that she was really proud of herself. She said, 'Before I did the Hypnobirthing Course I had no idea what a surge was for, I just thought is was a pain like you get when you are ill. After the course I really understood what the surge was for and actually that is was a positive thing – a positive energy. I knew the surge was my body working to birth my baby – it was for a reason, and a good one at that!'

This mum also told me that she did not feel any pain during her surges. She did, however, describe in great detail the sensations of her body opening and the power of her body had to move her baby down and out. She used words such as 'pressure' and 'heaviness' but she was very sure pain was not a word she would use to describe what she felt. Was there a connection between her confidence in her ability to birth, together with her understanding of the birthing body and her experience of birth? Of course, there has to be!

Chapter Five

The Pain of Childbirth

Pain is a word very commonly associated with childbirth. The debate about pain and childbirth draws many different opinions and is often an emotive subject.

Opinions vary too, from the idea that pain is inevitable or even necessary for childbirth to the idea that it is not natural to feel pain during childbirth at all. Some argue that it is an important contributory factor to the 'Right of Passage' that childbirth undeniably is (Leap, Anderson, cited by Downe, 2005). Others argue that the pain so many women experience is a throwback to the days when women and their offspring would have been vulnerable to the dangers of predators whilst giving birth and so the pain would be a signal to move to safety - a signal that they were about to birth.

The idea that pain is a signal to women to find safety has a certain logic but ignores the fact that a woman's body will send many other signals to her that she is birthing. Over the past few years I have met a significant number of women who have been very certain that they didn't experience pain during their hypnobirth, not one single one of these women said that they didn't know they were birthing or about to have a baby. Some have been surprised at the speed at which they birthed but all have described the distinct and powerful physical sensations they felt - often in great detail. They have described feelings of downwards pressure or a feeling of 'opening up' or 'a powerful force of nature' or such like descriptions. It is also important to note that none of these women saw their experience as anything less than amazingly phenomenal. To suggest that birth was any less a 'Right of Passage' for these women who describe their births in the most wonderful terms would be wrong.

A real case for pain being necessary for childbirth has never been made and if we consider the reasons why we sense pain in the human body it leaves no rational explanation as to why a BW would experience it.

Why do we feel pain?

It is widely accepted that there are two main reasons we feel pain;

1. Pain is a signal that something is damaged or wrong with our body and

2. Pain is a signal to stop or change what we are doing.

Considering this, it is not rational that a woman should experience pain whilst birthing. In the normal course of events there is nothing damaged or wrong with the birthing body during birth, it is carrying out a normal, natural bodily function. It's also worth considering that if there were something wrong during birthing, which of course can sometimes happen, how could a woman's body signal danger to her if she were already experiencing pain? Wouldn't it make sense that a woman knows she is about to birth by other signals, such as an urge to push or her waters breaking or by sensing the baby moving down onto the perineum, then if there was something to be concerned about, something damaged or wrong with her body *then* she would feel pain in order to recognise the danger.

Next considering the second point, if pain is a signal to stop or change what we are doing what would we stop or change? If the surges act in such a way as to open the neck of the womb and then push the baby out of the mother then there is nothing that should be changed.

Although the human body can be a quirky thing at times it does not make sense that the uterus would be the only muscle in the body that when it's doing the job it is designed to do (i.e. give birth) would experience pain. For example, if you use the muscles in your hands for gripping, carrying or holding, the muscles will work perfectly well and be very comfortable as they are designed specifically for these functions. However, if you were to stand on your hands the chances are that those muscles will become uncomfortable and even painful as, generally speaking, they are not designed to take the whole body weight.

"Ah but!" I hear you cry, "if I were to grip or carry something using my hands for many hours the muscles *would* hurt then, even though they might be doing the job they were designed for!" This is true. However, in my opinion, the pain felt by women during childbirth simply isn't the result of an overworked uterine muscle and this is why.

The muscles in the body can roughly be divided into 'voluntary' and 'involuntary' muscles. As they suggest the voluntary muscles are ones we can 'volunteer' or have a conscious control over and are controlled by the Somatic Nervous System. We think about moving our arm and it moves, we think about keeping our leg still and it stays still. The thinking part of our conscious mind has total control.

The involuntary muscles are the 'autopilot' part of our bodies and we do not have conscious control over them. Involuntary muscles include our heart muscle and bowel muscles. We cannot control our heart rate for by thinking about it and although some claim to be able to slow down their heart rate by conscious thought, generally speaking our hearts carry on ticking along whatever. Peristalsis is another good example of involuntary muscle action. Peristalsis is the wave-like motion of the bowel which moves digestive contents along the gut and is on the go 24/7. Again, generally speaking we tend not to be aware of this and don't have a conscious control over it either, in other words, it does its own thing.

Some muscles are both involuntary and voluntary such as the muscles used in breathing or blinking. When we are asleep and for much of our waking time our breathing carries on unconsciously but we can have a conscious control over our breathing too, choosing to take a deeper breath or hold our breath if we wish.

The uterus is an involuntary muscle. We do not have conscious control over it. The uterus will birth our babies whether we think about it or not - it just happens.

When the involuntary muscles in the body are doing the job they are designed to they do not hurt. Take the example of the heart. The involuntary muscle of the heart will beat over 2.5 billion times in an average lifespan and yet we hardly notice it. The only time we might experience pain in the heart muscle is if there is something wrong such as the chest pain felt during a heart attack, but a healthy heart will be free of pain. The big question is this, why would the uterus be the only involuntary muscle in the body that would feel pain when it is doing the job is was designed for even if it is doing that job for many hours.

Grantly Dick-Read said,

'No other natural bodily function is painful and childbirth should not be an exception.'

Chapter Six

Hypnosis, Hypnotherapy and Hypnobirthing

Hypnosis

The state of hypnosis is a natural state of being. Whilst we are awake our brain waves fluctuate as does our level of awareness. Take the average student sitting through a moderately interesting lecture. At times they will be totally focused on the lecturer and be fully consciously aware of the words being spoken and able to absorb their meaning. At other times their mind may wander, maybe they stare into space and daydream about what it would be like to be tucked up in bed or in the pub with their mates. Their level of focus or concentration will ebb and flow and during the times they drift off it's likely that they might feel that they have stopped hearing what is being said. This floating off or daydreaming is a natural state of hypnosis. The student allows themselves to dream and it feels pleasant. The conscious mind takes a back seat for a while and the subconscious is in charge.

The hypnotic state can also be a state of absorption. Everyone has had the experience of being very absorbed in a really good book or a film. As the storyline draws you in and fires your imagination the conscious mind becomes less active. It's possible to be so absorbed that you become much less aware of everything around you. Ever had that experience of being on a busy, noisy train and yet enjoying your book so much that the activity and noise fade right into the background? That too is a hypnotic state and also a very pleasant place to be.

The positive feelings attached to the hypnotic state means it is a state of mind that us humans will often seek out. Relaxing on a beach, listening to music, long distance running, listening to a story or watching a film can all encourage the state of deep relaxation. All of these leisure activities either encourage thoughts to become more fluid and free or for conscious thought to slow down, even pause for a while. Allowing the mind to become very absorbed is often something we enjoy as well, creative and leisurely pastimes such as playing an instrument, painting, reading, puzzles and even playing video games encourage this trance like state that we seem to find so pleasing.

So the hypnotic state (sometimes referred to as a trance) is a state of deep relaxation or absorption.

Purposefully taking oneself to a deeply relaxed place by using the imagination and breathing is referred to as self-hypnosis. Just take a moment to close your eyes and take a couple of extra deep refreshing breaths and then imagine yourself at your favourite place in nature. It can be anywhere, a beach, a forest, by a stream in a garden, on your allotment...anywhere. Imagine what you can see, hear, feel maybe even smell or taste, just imagine that favourite place. It's very likely that this simple exercise is relaxing and pleasant as you use your imagination it brings on a state of hypnosis.

If one person speaks to another using the right words in the right way so as to facilitate a state of deep relaxation or absorption then it could be said they are hypnotising them. If someone asked you right now to close your eyes, to take a deep breath, to relax your body and use your imagination to think of yourself on a warm and sunny beach and described that place in positive and sensory detail then it is very likely that you would become deeply relaxed. By following the words you would become hypnotised by them. It really is that simple.

Hypnotherapy

Hypnotherapy uses the hypnotic or trance state to introduce positive suggestions to the subconscious mind. Earlier I gave examples of how we naturally go into trance. But a trance or a deeply relaxed state can be induced as well. If a skilled person says the right thing in the right way to a willing participant then that skilled person will facilitate a state of deep relaxation within them. If someone encourages you to breathe slowly and deeply and then encourages you to use your imagination to drift off somewhere pleasant or asks you to focus your mind on something absorbing (like counting from 300 backwards) they can facilitate the hypnotic state. If they say the words in a gentle, calm and relaxing manner then you will find it easy to become deeply relaxed. The skilled person would then have induced a trance in you and this will open your mind to suggestion, you become more suggestible.

To make this clearer it is helpful to take some time to look at the mind and how it works, (well, what we know about the mind which is in reality very little). I'll try to put it in as much of a nutshell as I can and hope I don't do too much of a disservice to those who have dedicated a lifetime to understanding and describing the mind (Freud and Socrates to name a couple!) It is not my intention, either to give an overly detailed explanation here, just enough to make hypnotherapy and indeed hypnobirthing make sense.

The Mind

'*The mind is everything. What you think you become.*' Buddha

The Oxford English dictionary defines the mind as; 'the element of a person that enables them to be aware of the world and their experiences, to think, and to feel; the faculty of consciousness and thought'. Our mind and the thoughts and feelings within it make us who we are. If the body were a car the mind would be the driver. The car isn't much use without the driver and the driver gives the car meaning. Many see the spirit or soul as being linked or identical to the mind.

We all have a conscious and a subconscious mind. They are intrinsically linked and the boundary between the two is indistinct. For the purpose of understanding how hypnotherapy works, however, it is useful to think of the conscious and subconscious mind as slightly separate entities.

The conscious mind

Conscious thought's intangible nature mean it is classically difficult to define. It tends to be rational and analytical. We might think of our consciousness as our awareness or the 'here and now'. It might be described as 'the voice inside your head, I tend to call it 'the chatter' because that is what it is for me. Conscious thought will relate to the world around you, what you see, feel etc. and how you perceive it. Conscious thought can also give you a running commentary of what you are doing, not doing, need to do, are going to do etc. The conscious mind is more active more 'chatty' when we are awake and fully aware. As we relax or fall asleep the conscious mind slows down and becomes less active. The 'chatter' will fade away or even stop altogether as the conscious minds rests and takes a back seat for a while.

A few years ago my youngest son and I were walking together when suddenly he stopped, looked up at me with a look of wondrous surprise and said, 'Mummy! I can talk inside my head!' It was a lovely moment that I will never forget, he had become conscious of this conscious thought!

The Subconscious mind

The subconscious mind is the most powerful part of our mind and is said to account for around 90% of our thinking power. Subconscious thought is not limited by the physical body or the environment and this again makes definition difficult. The subconscious is made up of our emotions, creativity, imagination, spirituality, intuition and long term memory. The thoughts, feelings and behaviours that stem from the subconscious often feel like they happen all by themselves as we do not have a *conscious* awareness of them. Musicians will experience 'inspiration' as a melody just pops into their head as if from nowhere. The creative part of the subconscious has done the work for them and because of this they do not have a conscious awareness of it.

Ever had that experience of knowing you must have done something but really can't remember doing it? You're really looking forward to that cup of tea you made earlier, maybe you're busy and rushing around doing various chores or maybe you're very absorbed in reading or some other focused activity. You reach for the mug and as do you realise that it's completely empty, you stop, almost dazed for a moment. Where's it gone? I know I made it earlier so how could it just disappear? Quickly it dawns that you must have drunk it and simply not remembered doing so. You have drunk thousands of mugs of tea in the past and this one you drank totally subconsciously, you were on autopilot and so you don't have a conscious memory of it.

Drivers will often describe a similar experience especially when driving a very familiar journey. The driver arrives at the destination and as they pull up they are suddenly aware that they have no memory of part or even the whole of the journey. The route and the mechanics of driving are so familiar that they have become totally subconscious, a habit if you like and so the driver doesn't need the conscious mind to complete the task.

Habits are a really good example of the power of the sub conscious mind. Let's take the habit of smoking and let's call our smoker Henry. Now Henry is really clever, he has worked for many years as a surgeon and is at the top of his field. He is obviously very well educated and knows as well as anyone about the dangers of smoking and in case he might forget every time he takes out his packet of cigarettes the huge lettering shouts out 'SMOKING KILLS!'. So why does he still have that cigarette? Well his very powerful subconscious mind is in control here, and whatever thoughts, ideas and emotions are rooted there they're the ones driving the behaviour. The conscious rational and analytical part of this mind knows smoking is unhealthy, smelly and expensive but the unconscious thought thinks that in some way smoking will benefit him.

It's worth noting that the subconscious is associated with the autonomic nervous system. This part of the nervous system could also be viewed as our 'autopilot' as it controls bodily functions that happen all by themselves. Our heart beating, bowel moving, when we sweat or shiver etc are all controlled ultimately by the subconscious. The uterus too is controlled by the autonomic nervous system meaning birth truly is a subconscious act.

So how does Hypnotherapy fit into all this? How does hypnotherapy actually work?

Anyone seeking out Hypnotherapy will be looking to change something, a thought, feeling or behaviour that stems from the subconscious mind. Maybe a habit or a phobia or an anxiety for example. To help the client the hypnotherapist wants to appeal to the subconscious to change those unhelpful thoughts to ones that will benefit rather than hinder them. The hypnotherapist knows that when the conscious mind is active and full of busy thoughts that it can act as a barrier to the subconscious mind and can prevent it becoming open to suggestion. To encourage the subconscious to become more open to positive suggestions for change the hypnotherapist needs to facilitate the client into a state of deep relaxation (what you might call a trance) or deep absorption. Once the client is very deeply relaxed the conscious mind will slow down and become less active and less busy, it will take a back seat, as it were, and the subconscious mind will open up and become much more accepting of suggestions. In the case of hypnotherapy the suggestions would be positive suggestions for change that would benefit the client. The hypnotherapist might suggest to Henry the smoking surgeon, for example, that there are other ways besides smoking for him to relieve stress and that he will love his non smoking, healthy body.

The experience of these kind of hypnotherapy sessions can be quite an amnesic one which I think sometimes gives it a mystical feel. The subconscious hears and absorbs the words and suggestions but because the conscious mind is bypassed there is less of a conscious awareness of what was said. Henry during his hypnotherapy sessions might have felt like he didn't really listen to the words or even that he might have drifted off to sleep but almost magically he doesn't feel like smoking a cigarette. He's not consciously aware of why that is as the change has been a subconscious one.

Hypnobirthing as Hypnotherapy

Hypnobirthing works in the same way and could be viewed as Hypnotherapy for Birth. In previous chapters I have already discussed how crucial it is for the birthing woman to be relaxed and the deep relaxation that comes with the state of hypnosis is extremely beneficial. Hypnobirthing also has the added ingredient of positive suggestion, suggestion that birth can be gentle and easy and that a woman's body is perfectly capable of birthing all by itself.

Many women and their birthing partners using hypnobirthing to prepare for their birth will listen to a hypnobirthing CD or MP3 track. There are a number of these on the market with many Hypnotherapists and Hypnobirthing Practitioners producing their own. These tracks are usually about 20-30 minutes long and will guide the listener into a deeply relaxed or deeply absorbed place. They will say the right words in the right way which means the listener will find it easy to relax, the conscious mind becomes less active and so the subconscious mind opens up to accept suggestions. By listening to such a track the hypnobirthing couple will firstly practise and improve their ability to deeply relax but also they will hear repeated positive messages about birth which will sink down into the subconscious and become part of their thinking.

I have spoken to many people who have listened to tracks like these and almost without exception the experience is simply that the more you listen and relax the easier it becomes to relax. Hypnobirthing women will often say they notice how they become more deeply relaxed, and more quickly with repeated listening. We all have the ability to relax (that's for sure) but most people will find they benefit from practicing it, relaxation is a skill, the more you practise it the better you get.

The power of repeated messages is tried and tested. We've all had the experience of finding ourselves humming the jingle from an advert we've seen on the TV (even annoying ones!) or noticed how children might repeat the slogan from an advert for car insurance, even though they are be too young to know what car insurance is! This pattern of behaviour is no coincidence as advertisers know very well that if we hear something often enough it simply sticks in our minds, sinks into the subconscious and becomes part of our thinking. We won't, however be consciously aware of that process - it just happens.

Hypnobirthing harnesses the power of the subconscious mind, using all this to benefit the birthing woman, her birthing partner and of course the baby. By learning to relax and think positive thoughts about birth the BW and the BP avoid triggering the Fight or Flight reflex which means the birth can proceed without disturbance.

Chapter Seven

The Benefits of Relaxation

Research has shown that when a pregnant woman releases cortisol as a result of stress that the cortisol, a stress related hormone, will pass through the placenta and end up in the brain of the unborn baby. This research has also shown that stress in the mother during pregnancy can be linked to developmental problems, childhood obesity and even behavioural problems in the child. (O'Donnell, O'Connor, Glover, 2009). It stands to reason that if a pregnant woman regularly, deeply relaxes, then she must be benefitting her unborn child. As she relaxes and breaths deeply she will increase the blood flow through the placenta as well as release endorphins which will work to lower the cortisol levels. It is very common for pregnant women to report how active their babies are when they relax and breathe deeply, I am sure their babies are enjoying the relaxation too!

It is quite noticeable that babies born into the peaceful calm of a hypnobirth are unsurprisingly peaceful and calm themselves. Some parents and midwives are taken aback by just how quiet Hypnobabies (and waterbabies) can be. Some think that a newborn baby needs to cry and scream to initiate it's first gasp and to breathe using its' lungs but this is not the case. I have seen many babies born in water or into a quiet and peaceful room who have not cried and still have breathed without any problems. When a baby moves down the birth path slowly and gently the amniotic fluid that fills the lungs before birth will be squeezed out. This means the lungs and airways become clear so that air can move into them to inflate the lungs and so the baby will begin to breathe. Putting the baby skin to skin with it's mother will release a massive surge of oxytocin in the newborn as well as thermoregulate the baby (keep the baby at the perfect temperature) all of which helps to establish breathing (Unicef 2012). If the baby has these conditions at birth they will breathe without the need for any crying, tickling or (god forbid) a smacked bottom!

Newborn babies react to stimulus and are total barometers of what is going on around them, particularly at an emotional level. If their first experience is a startlingly bright, noisy place with people shouting and their mummy screaming of course they are going to feel tense or even threatened and they will cry. If they come from the secure peace and darkness of the womb to a dimly light and tranquil room to hear their mummy's familiar and calm voice right with them, then there is nothing to worry them. The transition has been so gentle they probably don't even realise they've been born!

Chapter Eight

The Womb and how it works

The womb (or uterus) is a muscular organ which lies inside the abdomen and near the pelvis. Inside a pregnant womb there is a thin membranous bag (the amniotic sac or membranes). The membranes are semi-opaque and quite thin but surprisingly tough. The sac is filled with water (the amniotic fluid or liquor) and the baby happily floats around in the water during pregnancy. At the bottom of the womb there is an opening or a neck called the cervix, often referred to as the neck of the womb. During pregnancy the cervix remains closed and will be around 3-4cm long. A mucus plug will sit in the opening of the cervix during pregnancy and this will act as a seal or protection - protecting the womb and baby from any potential ascending bacteria. During pregnancy the cervix will be firm to the touch - very like feeling the end of your nose in consistency.

The womb is made up, roughly speaking of three layers of muscle fibres. The inner layer comprises of circular bands of muscle which become closer together and more concentrated as they get nearer the cervix. (diagram 1). The middle layer is a network of blood vessels supplying the womb with its all important blood supply. The outer layer is made up of longitudinal muscle fibres which go up and over the womb (diagram 2).

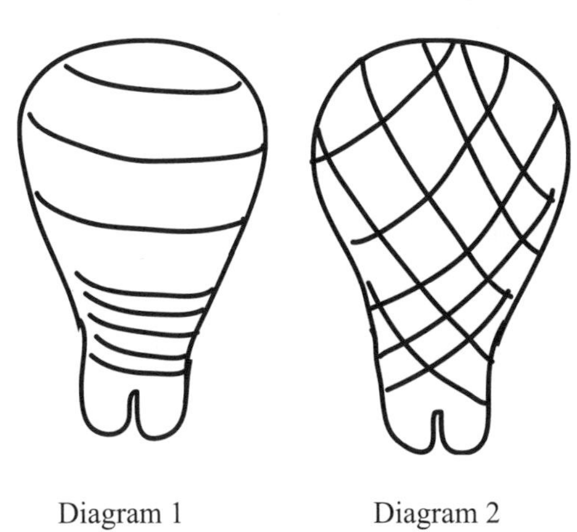

Diagram 1 Diagram 2

In the days or hours before a birthing starts the consistency of the cervix will change and it will become very soft to touch.

Then as the surges start the longitudinal muscle fibres will shorten or contract and, at the same time, the circular bands of muscle fibres relax. This whole action means the now soft, ripe cervix can be drawn up towards the womb. Every time this happens the cervix will get a little shorter or thinner (midwives call this effacement).

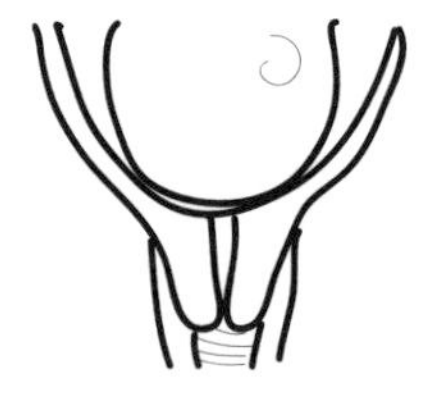

Cervix before thinning

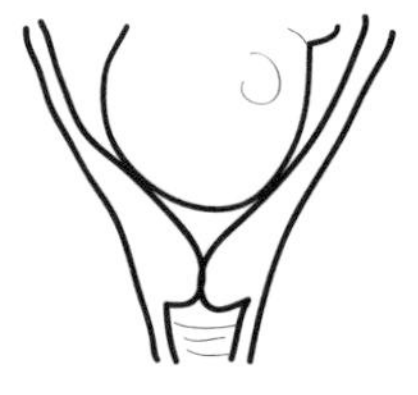

Cervix Beginning to thin

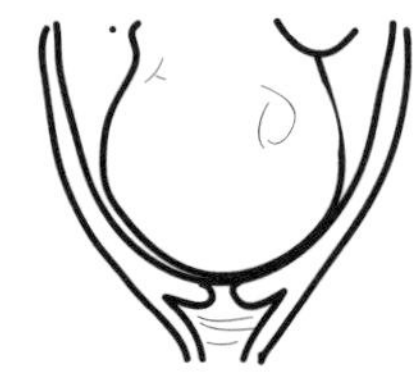

Cervix fully thinned out

The process of the muscle fibres of the womb pulling back the cervix will mean that, over time, the neck of the womb will go from 3-4cm long to as thin as paper.

The cervix is to be found at the top of the vagina, so if the BW or a midwife were to put a finger into the top of the vagina they would be likely to feel the top of the baby's head as it moves down into the vagina and the cervix in front of the baby's head. They would then be able to feel that the cervix was soft and how much it had thinned out by how long it was. So roughly speaking a cervix that is around 2cm long will be about half way through it's thinning stage. Depending on how much the cervix has thinned and opened they might also be able to feel the bag (the amniotic sac) bulging through the opening of the cervix. Over time, as the longitudinal muscles continue to pull back on the thin cervix it will be drawn further back and will begin to open. How much the cervix is open is measured by midwives in centimeters. For example it is generally accepted that for most women the active phase of birthing begins when the neck of the womb is opened or dilated to about 4 centimeters.

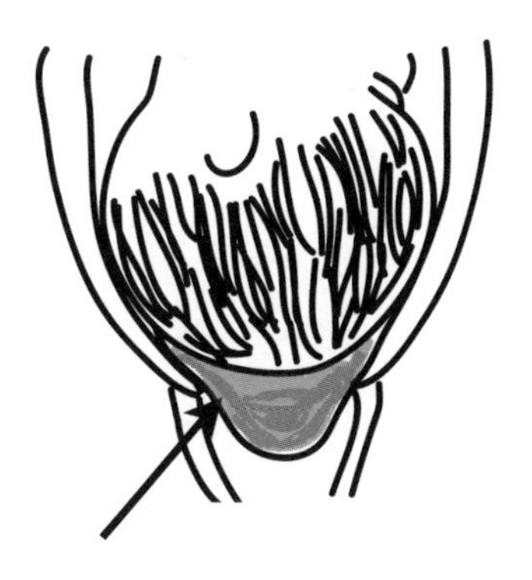

The amniotic sac bulges through the dilated cervix

As the baby moves down the birth path the water filled amniotic sac often bulges through the cervix. This is really helpful in encouraging the cervix to open up as it will stimulate the release of oxytocin.

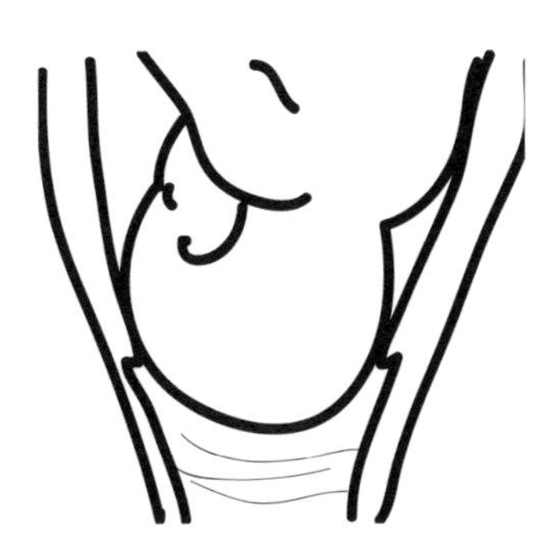

Fully dilated

After some time the muscular action of the surges will open up the cervix so far that it will all be drawn back towards the womb so that it is no longer in front of the baby's head. If you where to feel towards the top of the vagina at this point you would not be able to feel the cervix at all, just the baby's head and if the waters haven't broken, the water filled sac bulging in front. This is often referred to as 'fully dilated' or 10 centimetres dilated. All this means that there is room now for the baby to pass down the birth path towards the outside world.

As the neck of the womb becomes fully open the muscle fibres in the uterus not only contract and draw back but also begin to push downwards. This action is called retraction and means that each time there is a surge the womb it becomes a little bit smaller - it's already on it's way back to it's pre-pregnant size. This receding means that the womb will push downwards and, therefore, push the baby downwards also.

As the baby gets lower and meets the pelvic floor a reflex in the mother's abdominal muscles is stimulated. This is sometimes called the Ferguson's or abdominal reflex. It is very strong and the BW will find her tummy muscles join in all by themselves to help push out of her baby. The reflex is partially but not wholly involuntary. It will happen automatically if it is allowed. BW who are fearful or tense may resist the reflex and hold back the birth. Others may force the reflex, holding their breath, consciously pushing the abdominal muscles and straining downwards. I encourage BW to subscribe to the following mantra for this part of their birthing;

'I let it happen, all by itself, I listen to my body, it knows just what to do.'

The most marvelous thing about the abdominal reflex is that not only will it happen all by itself it will help to birth the baby at the perfect speed. The female birthing body is not only genetically programmed to birth but it also knows how to do it at the rate that is most beneficial to mother and baby. The rate at which a baby is born in a natural, normal birth is often surprisingly slow. The baby's head will very slowly and gradually slip out, rocking backwards and forth for a time and then as the baby moves out further very slowly appearing at the vulva a little at a time. This slow and steady birth will mean the infant has a gentle transition from the warm, dark, secure, womb. It also gives more time for the fluid to be squeezed out of the lungs as the baby moves through the birth path meaning that breathing in air will be easier when born. It is beneficial to the mother too as her baby passing slowly over her perineum means it is much less likely to stay intact and avoid tearing.

As the baby passes down the birth path and over the perineum the sensations felt by the BW whether they be of pressure, pushing, heaviness or bearing down will be very strong. Possibly one of the most important things to remember about this part of birth, though, is that it is involuntary and automatic or subconscious. The body at this point is on autopilot and the mother needs to let go and let it happen and trust it knows exactly what to do.

This part of birth is sometimes referred to as the birthing phase or the second stage of labour. During this phase women will often say, 'I *have* to push' or 'I need to push' expressing the instinctive power of that moment as they experience the irresistible urge to bear down. Women who are confident and trusting of their birthing bodies will welcome these sensations, recognising the awesome power or their body, understanding that that power is necessary to birth their baby and knowing it is meant to happen that way. It is essential at this point for the woman to really believe she can do it and that her body knows exactly what to do otherwise she is in danger of feeling overwhelmed and out of control.

In my opinion the following information is possibly the most important bit of knowledge a BW can have during the birthing phase. That is, that it is essential for the BW to understand that it *is* possible during the birthing phase to continue to breathe deeply and to avoid holding the breath and straining. It is possible to let all the powerful work continue as she breathes deeply. The breath may change (see page 71) but the deep breath should continue. The temptation in the less than confident woman is to let the downwards movement of the baby and the abdominal reflex become a conscious event and full of effort. This kind of forceful pushing is detrimental for several reasons. Firstly it is almost always associated with breath holding. During the birthing phase the surges can easily be 3 minutes apart and last for 1 minute or more. For the BW to be holding her breath every 3 minutes or so for a minute at a time can severely disrupt the respiratory cycle. In other words put simply she is not breathing enough. Some women who breath hold and push this way will literally swoon as their body becomes too low on oxygen.

Think for a moment about this breathing holding that is associated with forceful pushing;

1. An inwards breath is quickly snatched, the lungs are only partly filled with air

2. The breath is held during the forceful pushing, this might last 10-15 seconds or even longer

3. In order to quickly snatch another inhalation the remaining breath is quickly exhaled and the lungs are unlikely to be emptied fully

4. Steps 1 to 3 are repeated several times during a surge

Now consider the respiratory cycle and how we breathe naturally. To get a good amount of oxygen to the body we need to fill the lungs with air and use the diaphragm to breathe in (see Chapter Nine). Then as we breathe out we must do so fully to expel all the Carbon Dioxide (CO_2) as this is the waste product of the breath. If all the CO_2 is not exhaled it builds up in the system which can lead us to feeling short of breath and panicky as our body and brain sense the lack of oxygen.

When we breathe in fully and breathe out fully the body receives just the right amount of oxygen and expels the right amount of CO_2 to function properly. When birthing a baby the body needs to be allowed to function well and a lack of oxygen with a build up of CO_2 is the last thing it needs. Persistently holding the breath will mean the body doesn't have enough oxygen but just as importantly the baby will be affected too. The mother must breathe fully to oxygenate her baby via the placenta.

Forceful pushing, is sometimes called the Valsalva Manoeuvre (after Antonio Maria Valsalva a 17th-century physician and anatomist) and is still occasionally taught or encouraged by midwives and doctors as they think it may shorten the birthing phase and thus benefit the mother. Some BW initiate this type of forceful pushing themselves as they believe they are expected to push in this way as a result of suggestions given by births they may have seen on TV where puce faced women heave and strain whilst the midwife bellows 'Push! Push!' with great drama.

Several studies published between 1992 and 2009 (Nursing Times 2002, Martin 2009) showed that the physiological effects of Valsalva Manoeuvre can include: impeded venous return; decreased cardiac filling and output; increased intrathoracic pressure; affected flow velocity in middle cerebral artery; raised intraocular pressure; changed heart action potential/repolarization; increased arterial pressure; increased peripheral venous pressure; altered body fluid pH, which contributes to inefficient uterine contractions; decreased fetal cerebral oxygenation. In short the use of the Valsalva Manoeuvre has been shown to be detrimental to mother, baby and birth. The World Health Organisation, concluded that it is a dangerous practice and should cease. (WHO 1996)

The Royal College of Midwives as part of their 'Campaign for Normal Birth' (2012) suggest midwives do not instruct or direct BW with pushing in the birthing phase, they say,

'Evidence to date concludes that there are no data to support directed pushing in the second stage of labour and that spontaneous pushing, with a much shorter retention of breath (5-6 seconds maximum, compared with the 10 seconds of the Valsalva manoeuvre) has greater physiological effectiveness. Furthermore, the natural blowing out between breaths that occurs encourages her pelvic floor muscles to relax and reduces the risk of tearing.'

It should be mentioned that there are some rare occasions where it might be helpful to forcefully or consciously push in the birthing phase. A baby that is tired or struggling during birth but who is nearly born may benefit from an expedited birth. However, if all is fine with mother and baby and there is progress in the birth (i.e. the baby is coming out a little more with each surge) then there is no rational reason why a birthing woman should forcefully or consciously push her baby out.

The 'P' Word

There is an idea among some hypnobirthing teachers that the word 'push' should not be used in relation to the birthing phase at all. Some might even say that BW, BP and birth professionals should not even utter the word for fear it will suggest forceful pushing. I disagree. I think the word 'push' is a good descriptive word of the sensations that are felt in the birthing phase. The distinction that should be made is between the conscious and the unconscious push and great emphasis must be placed on the need to continue with deep breathing.

Once at a party I found myself chatting with a woman called Hope, who by pleasant coincidence had 'hypnobirthed' just 8 weeks previously. As with many woman who have used the techniques she was almost evangelical about it. She told me how she had been relaxed for a couple of days at home in the earlier part of the birth, arrived in hospital as the active phase of birthing was beginning (the cervix was 4cm dilated) and a few hours later had birthed her baby without the need for pain relief. Fantastic! Hope then looked down at her shoes and added in a hushed, confessional tone, 'I did push though, I just couldn't help it, actually that was the only bit I found hard!' Curious I questioned Hope further, how was it that hypnobirthing had helped her so much but the birthing phase wasn't so great. She described the strong automatic sensation of bearing down associated with the retraction of the uterus together with the abdominal reflex. That sounded perfect, I thought, so I questioned her further as to why, even though her birthing body was doing exactly what it needed to do she struggled at this point. She went on to tell me that when her hypnobirthing teacher had talked about this stage of birth she had stressed the importance of not using the word 'push' and she had said instead that the BW must 'breathe' their babies into the world. So when Hope experienced extremely powerful sensations of pushing, all be they instinctive, she thought that this must be wrong, that her body was doing something wrong and so what she was doing so naturally previously, then became difficult for her.

Breathing during this stage is good advice indeed but there is a danger in avoiding the word push altogether as some BW may feel that this means there will be no pushing at all. So when their birthing body spontaneously pushes they may feel negative and overwhelmed by the sensations.

When teaching hypnobirthing I prefer to be very clear about the difference between voluntary and involuntary birthing and between conscious and subconscious pushing. I emphasise the importance of breathing and just how powerful those sensations will be. Then the birthing woman can understand fully the process, be prepared for the power of her birthing body and stay in control and positive.

Chapter Nine

Breathing

Breathing fully and deeply is essential for feeling relaxed and for birth. Deep breathing has been shown to improve health, lower stress levels and aid relaxation. (Kaushik 2006, Cea 2010). Deep breathing will encourage the release of endorphins and oxytocin. Deep breathing will also oxygenate the body, the brain and in the case of the pregnant woman, the baby.

Inhalation

Modern living and stressful states tend to result in quick shallow breathing where the upper chest muscles are used and the lungs only partially fill with air. To breathe fully and fill the lungs with air the diaphragm must be used. The diaphragm is a dome shaped sheet of muscle that lies underneath the lungs.

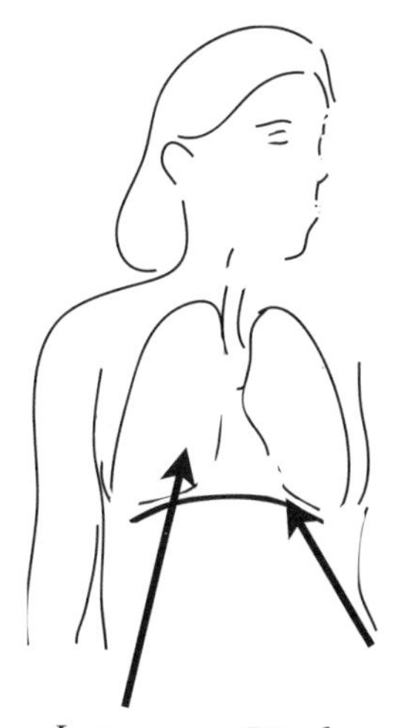

During inhalation the diaphragm flattens and the rib cage expands making space for the air to enter into the chest. It is essential for the diaphragm to flatten and move during inhalation for the lungs to fully inflate and fill with air. Diaphragmatic breathing is also beneficial as it will gently move or massage the internal organs. The liver, stomach and bowel that lie beneath the diaphragm will move with each deep inhalation increasing the circulation and relaxing the muscles. This can be immensely beneficial for sufferers of digestive disorders such as irritable bowel syndrome. As far as birthing is concerned to oxygenate the body and the baby as well as releasing endorphins and oxytocin is crucial.

When the diaphragm is used for inhalation the abdominal muscles join it. This type of breathing is sometimes referred to as abdominal or belly breathing. Placing a hand on the upper abdomen to feel the rise and fall of the tummy muscles is a good way to check that you are breathing using the diaphragm. Another technique is to place a flat, relaxed hand on the upper abdomen and then gently feel you are 'pushing' that hand away using the stomach muscles as you breathe in. Inhalation should be through the nose, audible and feel good, it may help to imagine you are standing on a beautiful, warm and sunny beach and breathing in the sea air.

Exhalation

The exhaled breath should be long and slow and smooth. The whole body should go loose and limp, like a rag doll. The exhalation is the time to release any physical tension, letting the shoulders sink down and the jaw to release and relax. As mentioned previously it is important on the exhalation to breathe out all the CO2 produced by the body as a result of respiration. For most people to expel all the CO2 means that a fairly long out breath is best to ensure you breathe out fully. As the body relaxes then it is easy for the mind to follow. Imagine you have just arrived home after a long and difficult day at work. As you sink onto your sofa you give a long and loud sigh maybe even blowing out as you exhale. As you do your mind also sinks down and relaxes, this is something we do quite naturally to aid relaxation.

Generally speaking it is better to breathe in through the nose and out through the mouth. The nostrils will warm, moisten and clean the air as it goes in. Breathing out through the mouth seems to come naturally to most during deep breathing. There is no specific reason to breathe out through the mouth, however, and some breathing techniques suggest exhalation through the nostrils. Once again I would suggest to do what comes naturally, feels easy and aids relaxation.

Breathing techniques

Breathing techniques are a way of focusing the mind on the breath to enable it to be full and deep. Many people find that focusing on a specialised way of breathing means it is easier to breathe well. Breathing techniques are commonly used where breathing fully is important such as yoga, pilates, singing, sports and drama.

There are so many different breathing techniques that it would be impossible to describe them all here. Some antenatal teachers including hypnobirthing teachers will prescribe certain breathing techniques to pregnant women, describing and teaching two or three techniques that must be used. This 'one size fits all' approach can be problematic because how we think about breathing will be as individual as we are. If you take a class of pregnant woman and teach one breathing technique it is very likely that a number of those women will not find that techniques suits them as it does not feel natural. There is a danger then that those women feel they cannot breathe correctly and that they have failed.

Every healthy adult, without exception, has the ability to breathe fully. How each individual achieves good abdominal breathing will be up to them. A hypnobirthing teacher should guide the hypnobirthing couple by giving different examples of breathing techniques so they can try these out for themselves during the class and at home. The couple should also be given reading material about breathing techniques and be encouraged to explore different ways to breathe fully and find what works for them. They will know a breathing technique is right for them when it brings about abdominal breathing and feels natural and relaxing. If a breathing technique requires too much effort and concentration and feels challenging then it is wrong and should not be used. Fundamentally if it feels good then do it!

Deep abdominal breathing can be just as useful for the BP as for the BW and should be practised by both. Most anxiety and stress will be accompanied if not preceded by quick shallow breathing. It is essential both for their own experience but also to be supportive to the BW that they remain calm and relaxed throughout the birth. Becoming practised at slowing down the breath and filling the lungs with air by regularly using a breathing technique can be incredibly useful.

With practice breathing fully can become second nature when used during birth. Relaxation and deep breathing are skills and like any skill if it is practised enough becomes a subconscious behaviour that requires little effort or thought. I suggest to hypnobirthing couples that they practise deep breathing for at least 15 minutes, twice daily.

It is not necessary to use a breathing technique for every single breath. In most cases the techniques are useful to initially focus the mind on the breath and once deep relaxation is achieved the breathing will become subconscious and carry on all by itself. However it is useful to refocus on deep breathing from time to time throughout the period of deep relaxation, this ensures the breathing remains slow and full. Some find that refocusing on the breath at regular intervals deepens the level of relaxation.

For some, using a breathing technique does not feel natural and makes them too conscious of their breath. Breathing is one function of the body that is both voluntary and involuntary. We can consciously start or stop our breathing, decide to breathe slower or quicker, but most of the time and when we sleep we do not breathe with the conscious part of our mind. It runs on autopilot. When we are in a deeply relaxed or hypnotic state our breathing will be automatic, this means the subconscious will be in charge and the breath will be deep and rhythmic (just like when we are asleep). There are those who find they can get into a deeply relaxed place easily, they don't have to think about it and quite often can't say how they do it. For those individuals using a breathing technique might be counter productive, making breathing feel unnatural and even causing them to feel short of breath. What was a natural, subconscious process becomes conscious and less natural. If this is the case there is no need to worry, someone who can skip straight to deep subconscious breathing and relaxation should not question how they do it but be pleased they can!

For the most part using a breathing technique to focus on the breath initially and then to refocus from time to time will be helpful. Focusing on a breathing technique can be useful as a way of staying calm and relaxed during a potentially challenging moment such as a surge or as a way of avoiding feelings of stress or fear. A few years ago a couple, Debbie and Mark, who had used hypnobirthing told me how important breathing was during their birth and in particular as they arrived at the birthing centre. They had stayed at home for the earlier part of the birthing and described a day spent relaxing listening to music with candles and massage. As the birthing became more active they had travelled into the birthing centre and as they arrived they had been asked to wait in reception so they could see a midwife. A very pleasant and smiling midwife arrived a few minutes later and explained to them that everything seemed absolutely fine and that they just needed to wait for a room to become available which would take half an hour or more. This was something that Debby in particular had not anticipated and she described how for the first time that day she began to feel out of control. The surges that had previously been perfectly manageable became painful and began to feel a little overwhelming. Debby, however, had enough knowledge and insight to understand what was happening. She knew that the wait in reception had distracted her, made her less relaxed and her breathing had become quick and shallow. She said she knew how important it was to breathe deeply and to relax and not allow the adrenaline levels in her body to rise. She knew she needed to encourage the release of endorphins and oxytocin. So she simply put her arms around Marks's neck and rested her head on his shoulder (a cuddle will stimulate the release of oxytocin and endorphins). Then she asked Mark to take some deep breaths. As Mark breathed slowly and deeply she followed his breath with hers - all she had to do was follow his breath. And as she did she noticed how the surges became manageable once again, she was aware of her body becoming more relaxed and felt she could now cope with the unexpected turn of events - and all with a deep breath. It didn't matter where she was and what was happening around her, the strength to carry on and the ability to relax had come from within her, she had used her internal resources to feel better. How wonderful to know that no matter what, you can still feel calm, relaxed and confident. Using hypnobirthing to avoid the Fight of Flight reflex means that birth is more likely to go smoothly but even if there are blips or unexpected events along the way the hypnobirthing couple can still be in control and maintain a calm confidence.

But I can't breathe deeply because my bump is in the way!

Many women, particularly towards the end of their pregnancy will complain that they are not able to breathe fully and fill their lungs with air. It can feel like their bump is in the way and taking up room in the chest. (It should be mentioned that any shortness of breath should always be checked out by a doctor or midwife as sometimes this can be a sign of anemia or other conditions that might need treatment). For many women this feeling is as a result of the baby sitting high up in the abdomen and against the diaphragm, therefore, it has less room for manoeuvre as it were. Often this is simply a question of allowing the baby to move downwards into the pelvis and away from the diaphragm. To encourage the baby to move down and into the pelvis and away from the diaphragm try the exercise below;

1. If you are sitting on a chair or sofa bring yourself towards the edge so that your feet are flat on the floor and about 30cm apart so that your feet are in line with your hips. A birthing ball is great for getting into the right position or try sitting back to front on a dining chair.

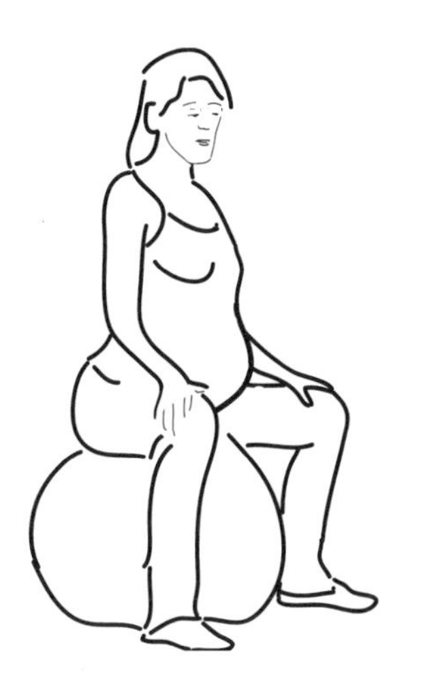

2. Get someone to have a look and check that your knees are lower than your hips - this will help to open the pelvis. If your knees are not lower than your hips raise your seating level with a couple of pillows.

3. Now make sure your spine is relaxed and straight and that you are slightly forwards, you might find it helpful to have a pillow or cushion on your lap for this.

Posture like this will encourage the baby to move into a good position and down into the pelvis and in most cases the pregnant woman will find this comfortable and will be able to breathe fully.

Described below are some ideas for breathing techniques. As discussed above it is by no means an exhaustive list but may be useful as a guide.

Balloon and bellows

As you breathe in imagine the abdomen is a balloon inflating, make sure the shoulders stay down and relaxed. At the same time imagine the rib cage is like a pair of bellows opening and making space in the chest for the air to be drawn in. There is no need to think about the mouth or the throat or even about breathing, just about the ribs and abdomen expanding, the air just happens to be drawn in as a result. As you let the breath out imagine the balloon gently deflating and the bellows folding and let the whole body go loose and limp.

Count the breath

Counting is very hypnotic. Hypnotherapists will often use counting as a method of refocusing the mind. The conscious mind can become pre-occupied with counting so that it becomes absorbed and less active allowing the subconscious mind to open up. Use the balloon and bellows technique as described above and then add a count of three for the inhalation and five for the exhalation. Note - the count should be at the pace that feels right for you.

The Golden Thread

Breathe gently in through the nose and then gently out through slightly parted lips. Imagine you are blowing out or spinning a beautiful, fine golden thread. Imagine the thread goes on and on until it finally falls over the horizon ready for the next in breath.

The Long Breath

Imagine as you breathe in that the breath starts at the fingertips, then moves up the arms into the shoulders, and then exhaling down the through the chest and into the abdomen and legs, and gently out at the toes. Take care to keep the shoulders relaxed.

Dropping a stone into a well

Imagine a deep well deep within you or deep within your abdomen. Then imagine that you are dropping a stone into this well as you gently exhale. Follow its path as it falls. Let the stone fall all the way to the bottom of the deep well. How long did the fall last? How deep did it fall? Where did it come to rest?

Hole in the Small of Back

This breathing technique is a useful way of taking attention away from the mouth, chest and throat if the breath becomes too conscious. Imagine a hole in the small of the back, through which the breathed air flows in and out of easily. Let all the focus be on the hole and that part of the back. Also imagine that the air being drawn in through the hole brings relaxation with it and that the air coming out of the hole takes any tension away with it.

Swing

Imagine a swing swinging with your chest and abdomen or if you prefer in your imagination. Pull back on the swing on the inhalation and on the exhalation gently push the swing and allow it to swing long, slow swings.

Waves or Tides

Imagine waves lapping onto the shore. Imagine the back and forth motion of the waves. Let your breath flow with the waves, in and out, let the waves and your breath find its own rhythm.

Bottle breathing

Imagine a bottle and let it sit gently within your abdomen. As you breathe in imagine the bottle filling with air or water and as you breathe out the level of air or liquid goes down with the out breath.

Rectangle Breathing

Imagine a rectangle. As you breathe in imagine the breath goes up one of the shorter sides of the rectangle and as you exhale let the breath go along the long side. On the next breath the rectangle is completed.

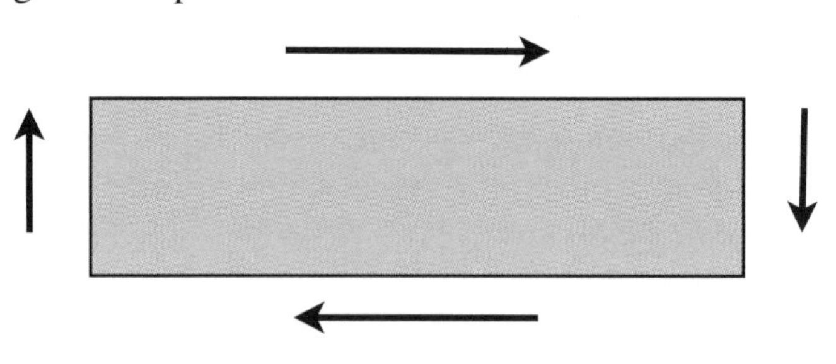

Birthing Breathing

As the cervix becomes fully dilated the muscle fibres of the womb will begin to retract and get shorter with each surge. This action causes the baby to move down the birth path and to birth. As all this incredible work goes on the pressure within the abdomen naturally increases and this in turn means there is an increase in pressure on the diaphragm. This increase in internal pressure can mean the exhalation can have a little more pressure with it too. When women are instinctively birthing they will very often 'blow' out during this part of the birth. I have been with BW who have exhaled with a long, low hum as they have breathed out or even an operatic style sustained note.

Blowing gently out through a relaxed mouth at this point during birth will avoid forceful pushing. It is almost impossible to forcefully push whilst breathing in this way as straining usually involves breath holding. If the BW is breathing deeply the birthing body will carry on physically all by itself, birthing at the perfect rate. Also there is the obvious advantage to continuing to breathe through the birthing phase, that is the oxygenation of mother and baby!

Blowing gently out through the mouth as the baby moves further and further down can be an external expression of internal sensation.

Breathing Technique for the birthing phase

1. As soon as the surge begins fill the lungs with air (consider using the balloon and bellows technique as described above)

2. On the out breath gently blow out with relaxed face and jaw.

3. Use a visualisation and imagine blowing bubbles or blowing a feather across the room in order to keep the face, mouth and jaw soft.

The following is a short script for during the birthing surges. If this verse is recited with a gentle, slow, relaxed pace it will be around a minute long and around the time a surge will take. The language in the verse is pertaining to the birthing phase.

(During surge)
Remember your body is perfectly designed to birth your/our baby,
Listen to your body, let go and let it happen,
Relax and breathe, breathing all the way out,
Let all your focus be in your head and face now, eyes gently closed, jaw relaxed,
Leave your birthing body to it's work now..it knows what to do and focus on the breath, breathing all the way out,
You can do it..you <u>are</u> doing it,
Breathe and relax,
Breathe

(In between surges)
Now let your breath go to a safe and natural pattern that's just right for you,
Jaw relaxed, shoulders release and relaxed
Just rest and breathe

Chapter Ten

The Birthing Partner's Role

Birth is a profoundly physical and emotional experience. For the BW to remain calm and relaxed during this time requires focus and concentration. Hypnobirthing women will often 'go within', get 'in the zone' or become quite trance or sleep like as a result. This peacefulness encourages the birthing hormones to flow and the birth to proceed without hindrance. The birthing partner and midwife should be considerate and respectful of the need for peace and calm in the environment and around the birthing woman. This may mean keeping noise levels to a minimum, avoiding unnecessary chit chat, keeping the lighting levels low and perhaps even keeping visitors away. A tranquil environment will mean the birthing woman will feel less distracted and more secure and, therefore, more likely to avoid the fight or flight response.

In the same vein it is also important to be considerate about the words and language that are used when communicating either in earshot of the BW but also when communicating directly with her. Positive supportive words spoken calmly will suggest confidence and relaxation and it is essential to avoid negative or anxious words which would only suggest fear and tension.

As a newly qualified midwife I spent a night shift attending the birth of a woman called Terry. Her birthing had been fairly protracted and yet she had the strength to carry on needing only a few words of encouragement. Although at times Terry expressed that her energy levels were low, her partner, Jay, didn't say anything but quietly rubbed Terry's back and legs for her and from time to time he made her tea with honey. Terry was strong and Jay's peaceful, supportive presence was enough for her. As my shift was coming to an end another midwife, arriving for the day shift came to take over. Now it so happened that this midwife had briefly met Terry when she had been admitted to the ward the day before. As she walked through the door she instantly recognised Terry and with a look of surprise exclaimed, 'Oh you're still here! You poor thing! You must be shattered!' I must point out that this midwife was a very pleasant, caring and hard working colleague. The words she spoke came from a place of care and concern but as those negative words landed on Terry's ears she physically slumped, her shoulders stooped and her head bowed down. Less than an hour later, just as I left for home, Terry was asking for an epidural because she felt she couldn't go on.

I feel the suggestion 'you *must* be shattered' became a part of Terry's thinking. 'I *must* be shattered, therefore I am.' Even though Terry had been birthing for over 24 hours and she had vocalised at times that her energy levels were low she had not expressed that she couldn't carry on or that she needed pain relief. Jay had said very little but had responded with gentle positivity, using massage, energising snacks and more than anything a quiet trust of Terry's strength, he never even once appeared to doubt that she could do it. It's a strong possibility that the day shift midwife's misplaced words sowed the seeds of doubt in Terry's mind and changed the whole nature of the birth.

During any birthing it is essential that the birthing partner and attending birth professional are mindful of keeping their words positive. Instead of saying 'Are you sure you can carry on?' much better to say 'Wow! You're amazing, you're so strong!'

Possibly one of the most insensitive comments I heard a birthing partner say was, 'God, this is going on forever! I can't believe you've not had an epidural by now!' The BW on the receiving end of this tactless statement answered in terms that are not printable here but her aggressive, defensive words were accompanied by tears of sorrow.

Most birthing partners, however, will naturally use positive affirming words, during birth. Simple statements such as, 'Well done! You're doing really well!' are positively affirming and supportive. Anyone present at a birth, however, needs to understand the power of suggestion and be careful to use relaxing and positively affirming language. The first rule is, if in doubt say nothing! What most BW want from their birthing partner is for them to be present and not just in the physical sense but a calm emotional presence. Being right there, ready to respond to requests and sharing the experience. A peaceful silence punctuated by gentle words of encouragement from a supportive emotionally 'present' birthing partner is usually enough.

Hypnotic Language

Being conscious of using positive language is important and birthing partners may take this to the next level by purposefully using hypnotic language to help induce a state of deep relaxation in the BW. Many hypnobirthing women find it particularly useful if their BP guides them to a deeply relaxed place by saying the right thing in the right way. Just as the hypnotherapist uses the right words said in the right way to induce a trance or state of hypnosis the birthing partner can do the same.

Hypnotic language will facilitate a state of deep relaxation or absorption. Hypnotic words often sound poetic and are soft positive words spoken in long flowing sentences. This way of speaking appeals to the subconscious.

It is always best to use permissive language too, using 'perhaps' or 'maybe' to suggest the experience rather than prescribe it. For some the mention of a hypnotherapist conjures up images of the brylcreemed doctor in his pin striped suit swinging his pocket watch and commanding 'You are now feeling veeeery sleeeepy...'. The problem with this kind of commanding language is that it can create oppositional thinking. For example, a client once told me that she was listening to a hypnotherapy CD which at some point stated, 'You are now at an ultimate depth of relaxation!' when she heard these words her reaction was to think, 'No I'm not!' and she therefore went on to worry that she was 'doing it wrong' and wonder why she wasn't at an 'ultimate depth of relaxation'. The result was that she stopped listening to the CD because it really wasn't relaxing at all! Perhaps she would have preferred the suggestion, 'and perhaps you become aware that your level of relaxation is becoming deeper', this suggestion is flexible and full of possibility. It is saying that you'll probably notice yourself becoming more relaxed but that there is no right or wrong.

Subconscious thought is nebulous, fluid and does not require the rationality of conscious thought. Everyone will have experienced the random nature of dreams or the hypnogogic state (that place somewhere between being awake and asleep) where the subconscious might throw out thoughts maybe about a penguin on the back of a camel and then suddenly about aunty Flo (except it's not aunty Flo) boiling her best shoes in a pan! Subconscious thought doesn't know the limits of the physical body and is not restricted by time or space. Unlike conscious thought it doesn't require analysis, patterns or even coherence. The kind of language, therefore, that appeals to the subconscious needs to reflect this, using the words 'perhaps you can be pleased to notice how each breath smooths and soothes away, and you can allow yourself to drift to that easy, comfortable place...' will mean whatever the subconscious wants it to mean, it is open and ambiguous, just like the subconscious.

This poetic, amorphous and permissive hypnotic language is sometimes referred to as being 'artily vague'. If the hypnotherapist says to their client 'your shoulders are now relaxed' that risks the client thinking 'no they're not!' but if they suggest 'maybe soon you will begin to notice changes and sensations in your shoulders and perhaps you have already noticed that they have begun to release and let go' they are much more likely to respond positively and accept the suggestion.

It is important that BP do not feel overwhelmed with all of this information. It is easy to feel the weight of responsibility 'what if I say the wrong thing? What if my partner can't feel or stay relaxed and it's all because I'm saying it wrong?' Firstly, remember that a quiet supportive presence is often enough. Secondly if there is any doubt as to what words should be spoken the BP should simply say 'breathe and relax' or 'take your time, I'm right here'.

The hypnobirthing mum should spend time preparing for her birth by practising breathing and relaxation techniques. The birthing partner should know that it is not completely down to them to induce the state of deep relaxation and confidence in the mother, it is more to reinforce and support it. The birthing partner will not be expected to take sole responsibility for the birthing woman's calm confidence, the BW must practise and prepare that for herself, the BP can then help to bolster and maintain the positive mindset.

Hypnotising as 'Mind Control'

Despite what stage hypnotists may lead the public to believe no one person is able to hypnotise another. A person can only go into a hypnotic state if they want to and will only allow themselves to go as deeply into trance as feels safe for them to do so.

I'd like to introduce you to Andy. Andy is a stage hypnotist and calls himself 'The Master of mind control!'. Andy is very popular, particularly in clubs and bars and frequently performs to hundreds of people at a time. Tonight he is appearing at a nightclub occupied mainly by stag and hen dos, it's busy and raucous. At the beginning of his show he firstly asks for volunteers, the more the better. Now Andy knows that it is very likely that anyone volunteering actually *wants* to be hypnotised. He also knows that the volunteers probably want the hypnotic show to go well and to make the evening an enjoyable and memorable one. There is a danger, however, that some of the volunteers want the opposite, maybe they are cynics and want to prove that hypnotism is a load of rubbish and that that they can't be hypnotised. So in order to weed out potential saboteurs and cynics Andy now 'hypnotises' the group by saying 'And now on the count of 3 you will feel veeeeery sleeepy and do excaaactly as I saaay! 1, 2, 3!' Andy will now observe the group. Some will instantly slump down into a hypnotic stupor immediately obeying his command, others may not respond at all and others may react but not quite so dramatically. Andy will already be focusing on the more willing subjects. Next Andy will ask all the participants to clasp their hands together and still observing the group will make lots of amusing suggestions that their clasped hands are stuck together with glue and no matter how hard they try they just cannot pull them apart. Again some of the group will follow these instructions perfectly and to great hilarity pull and pull at their hands but appear not to be able to pull them apart. The truth is they could easily move their hands apart if they really wanted to but they choose not too. At a subconscious or even conscious level the willing volunteers want their hands to stay together and maybe even be worried if they take their hands apart that the show and everyone's evening will be ruined. Andy then notices the members of the group who appear to have the most difficulty in pulling their hands apart and focuses on them for the rest of the show. Some nights he will only focus on one or two people other nights it might be as many as twelve or fifteen, it all depends on who he decides is most likely to participate. His skill is not in controlling the minds of others it is in making the right suggestions and be able to spot the most suggestible among the group.

Even Derren Brown whose whole career is based on persuading the public he can control the minds of other says,

'Despite the fact that to an onlooker (hypnotism) looks as if you've made someone go to sleep through some sort of hypnotic power, you start to realize that in fact you are only guiding your subjects down an easy path to what you want them to experience. You are not *making* them do anything.'

The birthing woman similarly, can only allow herself to be guided to a trance or deeply relaxed state if that is what she wants. The BP can help by saying the right thing in the right way, but she has to want it to happen. If she has practised breathing and relaxation then calming words from her birthing partner will undoubtedly be useful but she must initiate the process then allow her partner to help it along.

6 Easy Steps to being the perfect Birth Partner

Some birthing partners will feel confident and relaxed during birth and will naturally do and say the right thing. Most birthing partners use supportive words as a matter of course. For others who might be less sure here are six easy steps to being an effective and supportive birthing partner.

1. Keep the peace. As much as you can avoid loud noise or too much chat. Ever had that irritable feeling when someone near you is talking non stop? That irritation may be because the part of your brain that processes language is in the same part of your brain that controls the Fight or Flight reflex. So it makes sense that in order for the BW to avoid stimulating the Fight or Flight response it's probably best to avoid too much conversation.

2. Dim the lights. Darkness or dim light will stimulate the release of Melatonin. Melatonin is a hormone, sometimes called the 'sleepy' hormone. It is released into the body when it is dark and aids rest and sleep. Research shows that Melatonin can work together with oxytocin during birth to help surges be more effective and efficient. (Sharkey et al 2009).

3. If in doubt say 'breathe and relax' or 'take your time, I'm right here'.

4. Respond to any requests (e.g. for massage, food, a cuddle etc) calmly and without hesitation.

5. If in doubt say nothing! Silence really can be golden! But remain 'present' and close by. Enjoy sharing the experience.

6. Make sure you breathe fully as well. This will ensure you stay calm and relaxed so you can be supportive and enjoy the birth too.

A final note to birth partners is that they should resist the temptation to use a laptop or phone and to be connected to the internet or texting during a birth. Although there may be times when it seems nothing much is happening or when you may have to be patient and wait you should remember that attending a birth is a privilege and should command our upmost respect. If you are connected to the internet or you are having a conversation by text or phone you are no longer fully present, you are partly somewhere else. The birthing woman deserves and needs to know her birthing partner is there for her and just for her and that she doesn't have to share you with the world wide web!

Positively Affirming Language

If you see a child walking along a wall, wobbling and teetering and finding it hard to get his balance what might you say to him? You might be tempted to say 'Don't do that! You're going to fall!' but what does the child hear? Well they've just been told they're going to fall so they very likely will. As they tumble to the ground you might find yourself saying, 'See! I told you, you were going to fall!' but maybe they only fell because you told them they were going to! Perhaps it might have been better to say, 'Wow! That's clever how you're balancing up there. Now be really careful because it's high up, so come down now please.' This statement is clear and positive. You instill the child with confidence, suggesting they can balance so they are less likely to fall. You've told them what you want them to do rather than *not* do. If you say to the child 'don't do that!' it is not apparent what you *do* want them to do so they are left without direction. Saying ‘be careful and come down’ is stating what you *do* want them to do.

Unsurprisingly we tend to respond to positive language in a positive way. If an athlete trains hard for a race and puts everything she has into running that race and then comes in third place, would it motivate her to carry on if her coach said, ‘That wasn’t good enough! You only came third!’ or would she respond better to hearing, ‘Brilliant! You tried so hard and gave it your all and came in the top three! Keep going like that and you’ll be in first place before you know it!’

Now consider this in terms of the birthing woman. We have clearly established the need for her to be confident and to trust that her body can birth. Hypnobirthing women will have spent some time in preparation, building their confidence and learning to trust. During the birthing itself it is essential that she feels those around her are supporting her and also have confidence in her ability to birth. If her birthing partner tells her, “You’re amazing! You can do it! It’s brilliant that your body just knows what to do!’ then this will reinforce and support her self belief.

Chapter Eleven

Surges

The rhythmical work of the uterus during birth is often referred to as a contraction. The muscle of the uterus will shorten or 'contract' many times during birth in order to open the neck of the womb (cervix).

The word 'surge' has become widely used by hypnobirthers and midwives alike as a substitute for contraction. 'Surge' is a positive, descriptive word to describe the sensations and work of the birthing body. The body and uterus will surge with energy as each surge builds gradually, reaching a peak and then gradually fading away.

For women and men alike the word 'contraction' has a negative association that suggests a painful, difficult moment, something that will be overwhelming, out of your control and has to be endured. In contrast the hypnobirthing couple can celebrate the positive energy or the powerful and phenomenal surges that will birth their baby.

It is not a new idea to suggest the use of a more positive word than contraction to describe the work of the birthing body. Ina May Gaskin, often referred to as the 'mother of authentic midwifery' is considered to be one of the 'most famous midwives in the world'. In her seminal works 'Spiritual Midwifery' and 'Ina May's Guide to Childbirth' she uses the word 'rush' as an alternative to contraction. Ina May Gaskin has worked with birthing women for over forty years on a commune in Tennessee and holds legendary status around the world for her progressive, natural and spiritual approach to childbirth. Of note in 1992 a study (Durand 1992) of over 1700 births at The Farm concluded that that in low risk pregnancies births there were as safe as hospital births and often involved less intervention. An interview with Ina May in the Guardian Newspaper in 2009 said,

'During a Farm birth, you apparently do not experience pain, you have "interesting sensations to which you must pay full attention". You do not have contractions, you have "rushes"'.

In all her years of midwifery, Ina May has only ever known one woman who couldn't cope (there is no pain medication at the Farm, not even gas and air) and was taken to hospital at her own request. "We use a lot of tricks," she says. "We tell stories, we keep calm, we prepare the woman for how she's going to feel. Sometimes humour – even if it's gallows humour – is what works best."'

One of the most satisfying moments when teaching hypnobirthing is being able to say to pregnant women 'You're not going to have contractions! You're going to have surges instead!'. This is often met with a smile accompanied by a sense of relief!

Below is a Mantra for women to use in preparing their minds to think in a positive way about the work of the uterus during birth.

'I welcome each surge as it brings me nearer to meeting my baby. Each surge is a positive energy, working for me and my baby and my body knows exactly what to do.'

The pregnant woman should repeat this Mantra often. She could write it at the front of her diary or put it on the back of the toilet door or fridge door so she sees it often. This way the positive thoughts will sink into the subconscious and become part of her thinking.

When a birthing woman experiences surges during her birthing there will be an intensity of sensation. She will be very aware of the surges and their power. The surges need power and intensity to do their work and in most cases birthing women are very aware of the changes and movement that work involves. This is not to say that the power and intensity must be overwhelming or unmanageable or even painful. Far from it, with positive thinking, relaxation and knowledge the birthing woman can marvel at that power and let it work for her.

It is important during a surge that the birthing woman does not respond in a negative way to the intense and possibly new sensations that she is experiencing. I have witnessed too many women who, as soon as they were aware of a surge starting hold their breath and tense their bodies and literally 'brace' themselves - ready for impact! It is clear how important it is to continue to breathe well throughout birth and particularly during a surge. It is also important to keep the physical body free of tension. The surge itself may be felt as a pulling, tight or heavy sensation and it is essential that the rest of the body doesn't respond in a negative way to these sensations by tensing the shoulders or screwing up the face etc. Breathing fully and keeping the body relaxed during a surge will have many benefits. Firstly the obvious benefit of oxygenating the body and the baby. Secondly when the body remains relaxed there is no energy wasted in unnecessary tension. When the birthing body is fully relaxed the energy is conserved for the birthing part of the body where it is needed the most.

Techniques for Surges

The following are some techniques to stay physically relaxed and mentally calm during a surge.

Breathing and Counting

1. As the surge begins breathe all the way out by gently and quickly blowing through the mouth.

1. As the surge builds breathe in deeply through the nose, make the breath audible, so the breath can be heard moving through the nasal passages. As you are breathing in use the balloon and bellows technique (see page 68).

2. As you breathe out imagine a wave of relaxation moving from the top of your head and then all the way down through your body, right down to the end of your toes. Allow the wave to relax each and every part of your body as it moves down.

3. As you breathe out count slowly ‘5 and 4 and 3 and 2 and 1’.

In this technique the focus is on the breath and it enables the BW to continue to breathe fully throughout the surge. Also the focus is on keeping the body relaxed and free of tension.

Partner technique for during surges

1. The hypnobirthing couple stand together, facing each other, the birthing partner gently holds the Mum's hands as in the illustration below.

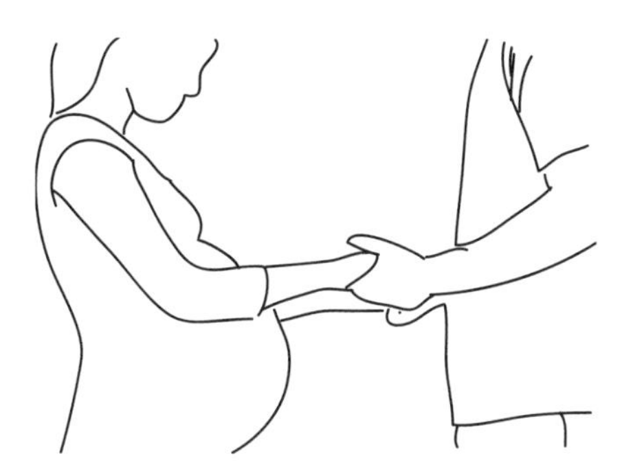

2. The hypnobirthing mum then lets her whole body become loose and limp and lets the birthing partner take the whole weight of her arms. The birthing partner should really feel the weightiness of her arms.

3. As the surge begins the mother breathes all the way out by gently and quickly blowing through the mouth.

4. As the surge builds she breathes in deeply through the nose, making the breath audible, so that breath can be heard moving through the nasal passages, using a breathing technique such as the 'balloon and bellow' technique (see page 68). At the same time the birthing partner reminds the mother to breathe fully by saying 'breathing all the way in' or 'as you breathe in bring that breath to our baby'.

5. As the mother breathes out the birthing partner gently raises the her hands and arms by about 6 inches. At the same time the birthing partner says, 'let me take the weight of your arms' or 'release and let go'. As the BP does this the mother must give over the whole weight of her arms to her BP.

This technique focuses on deep breathing and remaining relaxed. To allow another person to completely take the weight of your arms can be trickier than you might think and some couples need time to practise this. Allowing the birthing partner to take the weight of the arms works on two levels. Firstly the arms, hands and shoulders are common places to carry physical tension and for some it can be difficult to release the tension here. By raising the arms slightly and then letting them rest fully on the BP's hands, the hands, arms, shoulders, neck, chest and upper back will all release and relax. Secondly to allow someone else to take the weight of your arms requires you to 'let go' mentally as well as physically. To 'let go' physically, mentally and emotionally is necessary to birth in a relaxed and confident way. Letting go by giving the weight of your arms to another is a similar mental and physical process.

Chapter Twelve

Hypnotic Scripts

A hypnotic script is a written transcription of pre-prepared hypnotic words or a hypnotherapy session. Many hypnotherapists will only make notes when meeting a client for a hypnotherapy session and then use their experience and subconscious to find the right therapeutic words. At other times they might prepare a script, for example, to share with colleagues, facilitate group hypnosis or even sell to other hypnotherapists. Scripts can be useful for trainee hypnotherapists so they can learn what makes up a good hypnotherapy session and what kind of language is useful.

Hypnotherapy sessions are often structured with an Induction at the beginning, where the client is guided into trance, this is often followed by a Deepener, where special techniques are used to deepen the level of relaxation. After this the hypnotherapist might introduce some Post Hypnotic Suggestions - positive suggestions made whilst the client is in trance. Hypnosis scripts are often structured in this way as well.

As part of a hypnobirthing course the couple will be taught how to use a hypnobirthing script, then at the birth the BP can read it to the BW to help her to relax and feel confident. It seems particularly useful if the script is the transcript of the CD or hypnobirthing audio track that they have been listening to in preparation for the birth.

When a hypnobirthing mum listens regularly to a hypnobirthing audio track she will become very familiar with the calming and affirming words. Even if she feels she doesn't hear or remember the words because she drifts off into deep relaxation she will have heard them on a deeper, subconscious level. So subconsciously the whole thing will become very familiar. The more she listens the more she will associate the words with deep relaxation and feeling positive about her birth and, therefore, the words become a strong trigger (or anchor) for relaxation. If the birthing partner reads these familiar, calming words the effect can be fantastically powerful. For the BW this means her birthing partner is there, right with her and saying the right thing in the right way. I have attended hypnobirths where the partner reading a hypnobirthing script has been everything and all the BW has needed.

For the birthing partner too reading a hypnobirthing script can be a very relaxing. To read a script in the right way the BP needs to be calm and relaxed themself, it simply works better if the words are spoken by a calm and relaxed person. We tend to absorb and take on the mood of others, between humans there is almost an osmosis of emotion between us. We can find ourselves laughing just by hearing another person laugh even if we don't know what they are finding funny. Be near a person who is calm and confident and it is likely that some of that calm confidence will rub off. Be near by a calm confident person using calming and positive language and it would be very hard not to feel relaxed!

How to read a Hypnobirthing Script

Before reading a Script the birthing partner should check they are breathing deeply and that their body is free of tension. It's often helpful to shake out the hands and arms and take a deep breath before beginning. The pace and tone of the words should remain gentle and calm throughout, gentle words of support whispered in the ear. At many births birthing partners will naturally do this anyway, they instinctively know to be close by.

During a hypnobirthing course couples should be given some time to practise reading a hypnobirthing script. I have noticed that for some couples reading a script seems perfectly natural and easy, maybe they have been used to reading to each other for relaxation and leisure already. For other couples it is new and different, it's not unusual for a little nervous, self conscious giggling when first trying it out. Most couples will find that the self consciousness or giggling passes as they practise more and it all becomes a familiar and natural way for them to prepare for the birth together.

Chapter Thirteen

Visualisation

Visualisation or mental imaginary uses the subconscious in order to have a mental rehearsal for anything we might need to prepare for. For example the breathing technique called 'Bottle Breathing' (see page 70) uses visualisation. To use the technique you need to visualise or imagine a bottle filling and emptying as you breathe in and out. As you visualise the image of the bottle you will find it easier to focus and your conscious mind will become less active resulting in the breathing becoming more focused.

Visualisation can also be used to profoundly influence the way we think and behave.

A well known study which partly used visualisation took place in the 1980s where Russian Scientists looked at performance outcomes for Olympic athletes based on physical and mental training ratios.

Group 1 received 100% physical training;
Group 2 received 75% physical training with 25% mental training;
Group 3 received 50% mental training with 50% physical training;
Group 4 received 75% mental training with 25% physical training.

Group 4 had the best performance results and the Soviets concluded that 'mental images can as as a prelude to muscular impulses.' (Scaglione et al 1993)

It has become widely acknowledged in the world of sports and sports coaching that mental rehearsal, imagery or visualisation will enhance performance. Footballers will be coached to imagine the ball going into the back of the net before to taking the penalty, golfers are taught to imagine the path and flight of the ball before they take their shot. For hypnobirthing the benefits are clear. If a pregnant woman spends a significant amount of time contemplating her birth in positive terms then those positive visualisations will become part of her thinking and how she actually feels about birth. If her expectations for her birth are that it will be natural and easy then it is likely to be so.

You may have heard the term 'self fulfilling prophecy'. A self-fulfilling prophecy is a prediction that causes itself to become true, by the very terms of the prophecy itself. Our expectations can change and shape our behaviours and, therefore influence outcomes. A good example of this is a famous study where teachers told random students that they were "going to blossom". The results of the study showed that, those random students did significantly better (Rosenthal, 2003).

How lovely to think that just by using the power of her mind and imagination the pregnant woman can influence not just how she feels about birth but even the birth itself!

Visualisation is simple and easy to do, all you have to do is use your imagination and anyone can do that. How we visualise will be as varied as we are. If you are naturally a very visual person you might find you can imagine any scenario in full 3D colour but it's fine if you can't actually see it in your mind's eye. If you can sense it or feel it, imagine it or just hear your voice describe it then that's right for you and it will be real for you. There is no right or wrong to visualisation, it's whatever works for you and should feel natural and easy.

You can visualise anywhere, anytime. It's always a useful tool to have if you are in a situation that is stressful or boring. I suggest to women attending my hypnobirthing classes that they visualise their perfect birth as often as they can - on the bus, during their coffee break or in the queue at the post office! I suggest they use deep breathing and visualisation to feel calm and relaxed in any situation which might be stressful but they don't have much control over. Sitting waiting for an antenatal appointment can be the perfect time to practise. Imagine now you've been waiting a while and have no idea how much longer you'll be. You don't have any control how quickly you'll be seen so you decide to make the most of this otherwise empty time. You close your eyes and begin to dream. You imagine yourself at your birth. Everything is going just as you had wanted, you feel great, look amazing, everything is peaceful and everyone is calm. A perfect birth.

I also suggest that when visualising a good birth that women don't make the imagined scenario too specific. If a pregnant woman spends a good deal of time imagining herself floating serenely in the pool and then, for whatever reason, she finds she is unable to use the pool during her birth there is a danger she will feel that nothing has happened as she planned. Instead I would suggest visualisation should be about a general sense of peace and calmness in the birth, everything going smoothly and about feeling fantastic and in control. Of course there may be some detail of where you are and who is with you etc but it's best to have a sense that no matter what, no matter where you have the ability to remain calm, to breathe deeply and to feel confident and in control.

Hypnobirthing is about connecting with and developing your internal resources or your inner strengths. Women have an innate and instinctive ability to birth their babies all by themselves and without complication. A good number of women get into difficulties because they don't think they are able to do it and their body isn't able to birth. It is common for women during pregnancy to become very fixed on the circumstances of their birth, desperately hoping their favourite midwife will be on duty or that they will be able to birth in a certain birth centre or hospital. They may write a long and overly detailed birth plan outlining what should happen in any circumstance. They are feeling out of control and try to get a grip by controlling their surroundings and their circumstances. Hypnobirthing women of course will have preferences for their birth which may include to birth at home or in water. However they also have the powerful inner knowledge that no matter what path their birthing takes they have the ability to remain relaxed and calm whatever and wherever. This calmness brings with it a control and clear mind which is so essential for a gentle birth. The blind panic or fuzziness that comes with fear is replaced by a calm clear control and all this comes from within.

Chapter Fourteen

Anchors

Couples using hypnobirthing can make good use of anchors to feel calm, relaxed and confident during birth.

An anchor is any physical association with a feeling. It is anything external that triggers a feeling or emotion because we have an association with or a memory of it. Anchors can be positive or negative but for the purposes of hypnobirthing positive anchors are used. An anchor can be something we hear, see, smell, taste, feel or touch. Have you ever had that experience were you turned on the radio to hear a track playing and it instantly and immediately took you back years and years to a very certain time and place? That music was an anchor to those memories and it's very likely that one of the strongest elements of that memory was how you were feeling at the time. So the music not only anchored the memory of where you were or who you were with or what you were wearing it will have anchored your mood, feelings and emotions too. If as a child you had your head stroked or back rubbed as you fell asleep you would probably find it very relaxing now. The physical touch reminds you of how you felt at that time.

During the preparation for birth it is useful for the mother to practise deep breathing every day. By doing this she will become skillful at breathing fully and a deep breath will become an anchor for relaxation. She will associate breathing fully with calmness and relaxation and those feelings will be anchored to the breath. At the time of her birthing a simple deep breath will then easily bring those feelings of calm and peace.

A hypnobirthing audio track can also anchor feelings of calm confidence. The hypnobirthing couple are encouraged to listen to such a track regularly in the weeks and months leading up to the birth. The words and music become very familiar and very much associated with comfort and relaxation. The positive suggestions heard in the hypnobirthing track will sink into the subconscious and become part of the thinking and therefore the words anchor feelings of trust and confidence. For many hypnobirthers a hypnobirthing track becomes such a powerful anchor that even the process of putting the track on and listening to the introduction is enough to induce feelings of calm.

Technique for anchoring feelings of calm confidence during a surge

This technique can be used with the couple facing each other or with the birthing partner sitting or standing behind the birthing woman.

1. The birthing places their hands on the outside of the BWs arms close to the elbows or on the pregnant tummy.

2. As the BW breathes in the BP sweeps their hands up the outside of the BWs upper arms or up the tummy toward the shoulders at the same time saying, 'I feel relaxed calm and confident'.

3. As the BW breathes out the BP places their hands on the BWs shoulders and applies very gently pressure at the same time saying 'I am looking forward to meeting my baby'.

4.During the next breath the BP should move their hands down the upper arms back towards the elbows or back down the pregnant tummy ready to start this again. At the end of this breath the hands should be ready again at the elbows or bump to repeat from step 1.

This technique will anchor the physical touch of the BP, the sweeping up of the hands and the gentle pressure on the shoulders, to feelings of calm confidence. The more it is practised the more the mother will associate it with positive feelings as the anchor becomes stronger.

Finger and thumb anchor

1. Make sure you are comfortable before you begin, sitting is best with your legs uncrossed and hands lying loosely by your side.

2. Take a couple of deep breaths and close your eyes.

3. Spend a few moments visualising yourself at your birth. Everything is going just as you had wanted, you feel great, look amazing, everything is peaceful and everyone is calm.

4. Keep this image with you, let your whole body relax and repeat the following mantra in your head;

'I am a worthwhile person and I love and approve of myself'.

5. As you continue to visualise and repeat the mantra press the finger and thumb together on each hand.

6. After a few minutes give yourself permission to finish and move back to the present, take another deep breath, have a stretch and remind yourself of where you are and what day and time it is. You may notice how those feelings of

calmness and comfort for some time even after you have finished.

This exercise will anchor feelings of confidence to the physical act of pressing the finger and thumb together. This simple gesture will hold a memory if it is repeated several times. If the BW has practised this then she will be able to trigger feelings of calm confidence anytime, anywhere, quickly and easily.

Chapter Fifteen

Building Confidence, Dispelling Doubt

Pregnant women and their birthing partners should be able to approach their birthing full of confidence and trust. They should understand that birth is a fundamental function of the female body. A newborn baby girl is born already with around 1 million eggs in the ovaries and although they lie dormant until puberty it is an indication that the female body is perfectly designed for reproduction. Birth is completely automatic and even with all the technology and intelligence in the modern world we still really don't know exactly how it all works. What we do know is, that if a BW feels safe, calm, relaxed and confident her birthing body will know exactly what to do.

Fear is a word that is so often connected with birth and women preparing for birth will have differing levels of fear. Each individual's background, education, family dynamics, personality and personal experiences will shape their thoughts and ideas about birth. At the beginning of each hypnobirthing group I always ask couples to introduce themselves to each other and, if they are happy sharing it, to talk a little about their pregnancy, their preferences for birth and why they chose hypnobirthing. In most cases there is at least one couple in the group who's reason for attending is because they are terrified of birth and want to change that. Of course not all those attending are terrified, others will be excited about birth and keen to experience it in order to get their baby. It is very unusual, however, for someone before they have learnt hypnobirthing to be free of all fear of birth. Some women who might be confident in their ability to birth still worry about losing control and being subjected to unnecessary intervention. Others might have concerns that on the surface appear minor such as worrying if their partner will be able to get home on time from work once their birthing begins. There may be anxiety about life after giving birth and becoming a parent or even financial worries. Whatever the worry, fear or concern it is essential for the process and experience of birth, that these doubts are cast aside. Any fear, even a small niggle, might hold back the BW and make her reticent to 'let go'. Holding back mentally or emotionally will inevitably mean the physical body holds back too.

A few years ago I met a bright and vibrant woman called Olivia who came to learn hypnobirthing. She was a natural positive thinker and when I met her I was struck by how excited she was about the birth, having a baby and about hypnobirthing. Her partner Eric was equally enthusiastic and was very keen to be a supportive and useful birthing partner.

Olivia and Eric grasped the ideas of hypnobirthing easily and took it to their hearts, they fully appreciated the philosophy and wanted it to work for them. From time to time, whilst talking about their plans for their birth, Eric would mention his mum and it became clear that he and his mum expected that she would be at the birth. Every time Eric brought this up, however, Olivia's face would visibly drop and her eyes would become dull and serious. I asked Olivia how she felt about Eric's mum being at the birth as the change in her body language was so noticeable whenever it was mentioned. When questioned Olivia verbalised that she thought it was a good idea to have an extra person there to support her but also to support Eric too. As they finished their course they seemed upbeat and excited, they enjoyed practising the techniques together and felt they had already benefitted from learning to relax.

Several weeks later I received a phone call from Olivia. She still hadn't birthed her baby and she was a week past her due date. Although she wasn't concerned about being overdue she was worried about the possibility of induction of labour as her midwife had recommended that she should be booked in for this within a few days. As we discussed Olivia's options I mentioned the idea that some women might 'hold on' to their pregnancy subconsciously or on a deeper level. This might be because they are enjoying their pregnancy so much or because they are afraid of moving on to the next stage of being a parent or even afraid of the birth itself. It is still not fully known what actually stimulates a woman's body to begin to birth but it's likely that a release of oxytocin is necessary. Fear, stress and anxiety will all suppress the release of oxytocin and so it's possible that some women's births are delayed because they are fearful or stressed for whatever reason. As I began to put this theory to Olivia she started to cry. I hesitated - had I said the wrong thing! 'It's Sheila!' came the voice down the phone. I paused, 'Sheila?'. Olivia didn't reply immediately but I could hear her gentle little sobs, I waited. Finally Olivia said, 'Sheila - my mother-in-law. She's coming to the birth...and...well she's so lovely..I feel bad..'

Olivia went on to say that although she loved Eric's mum and valued her support she was worried about feeling exposed in front of her. She wasn't worried about birthing with Eric there or the midwives but her mother-in-law felt different. 'Why don't you tell her?.' came my reply, but Olivia felt she would be letting Eric and Sheila down by divulging how she felt. I reminded Olivia that it was her birth, no-one else's and if she was to feel truly safe and relaxed then she needed to know her birthing companions were there just for her and her alone. Olivia mused on this but she still wasn't sure what to do.

I knew that Olivia's anxiety about being exposed in front of her mother-in-law was rooted in her subconscious. She was probably unaware of why she felt that way or where those emotions stemmed from. Perhaps it was an idea passed onto her as a child or messages she had received from friends, family or the media as she grew up. Why she reacted in the way that she did was unclear as it was a result of subconscious thought. As those thoughts and ideas rooted in the subconscious had become part of Olivia's thinking I suggested that hypnosis was the best way to change them, Olivia agreed. I went through with her the 'Building Confidence - Dispelling all doubt' exercise as detailed below and Olivia said she would try it straight away.

It was six months later when I heard from Olivia again. I received a beautifully scripted hand written birth story and a completely unnecessary apology about her taking so long to send it! Reading the birth story gave me goose bumps as she described a beautiful, comfortable, gentle home birth in just over 8 hours. She did not mention our last conversation but she did not mention her mother-in-law either. She mentioned how fantastic Eric's support was and how the midwife was blown away by the calmness of the birth. I can only presume Sheila wasn't there or if she was, Olivia had come to terms with her fear. Either way it didn't matter, Olivia had had her perfect birth.

During a hypnobirthing course the couple should be taken through a Building Confidence and Dispelling Doubt Hypnosis session. The session lead by the hypnobirthing teacher will use Hypnosis to release any fears or negative thoughts about birth and at the same time to build and bolster confident thoughts.

This is something that should be done in a safe and supportive context such as a hypnobirthing group or a one to one hypnobirthing session.

If you find yourself imagining birth in a negative way or have a mental image or 'film' playing in your mind that is playing out any fears of anxieties about your birth try this exercise to quickly change the negative to positive.

Important note: This exercise should not be undertaken if the negative thoughts and ideas are traumatic. It is intended as a way to dispel doubts, fears or negative thoughts that may arise during the preparation for birth. If there are past traumatic experiences or extremely challenging and difficult thoughts and emotions you should speak to your GP who may refer you to a mental health specialist who works with post traumatic stress disorder or a qualified hypnotherapist.

1. Sit comfortably and close your eyes. Spend a few moments focusing on your breath. Take a couple of extra deep refreshing breaths.

2. Now, in your mind's eye, imagine that situation that is causing you to feel anxious or doubtful. Make the image very vivid, see it in full HD and make all the colours really bright. Make the scene very lifelike so it fills your whole vision. It might help to think of the scene on a big flat screen or like it is being projected into your mind. It may help to add scenery or other people to make it more lifelike. We're going to call this image 'moment of doubt'. Now take the 'moment of doubt' image and put it to one side in your mind.

3. Now for something more positive. This time you are going to create an image of your perfect birth. Again make it as

vivid as possible with sharp images and vivid colours. Make sure you look really relaxed and happy. Everyone around you is totally relaxed and everything is just as you hoped it would be. We'll call this image 'perfect birth'. When you connect with the feelings of calm confidence in this picture enjoy those feelings for a moment, then in your mind's eye see that image shrinking, and becoming smaller and smaller, with the colours getting duller and muted, until you are left with a small black and white picture the size of a postage stamp. Now put this image to one side in your mind just as you did the first image.

4. Now, pick up the 'moment of doubt' picture, and just like before make sure it fills your entire vision, and that it is just as life-like as before, but this time there is a small yet very important addition. The small, black and white 'perfect birth' postage stamp sized picture is now tucked into the bottom left-hand corner.

5. When you have that all clearly in your mind's eye, just say to yourself: 'S-W-I-S-H', (almost make the word melodramatic a really big S-W-W-I-I-S-H) and at the same time change the two images over in your mind so that the 'perfect birth' picture becomes the bigger colour picture and the 'moment of doubt' shrinks to the size of a postage stamp tucked into the bottom left-hand corner, becoming black and white as it does so.

6. Enjoy this for few moments.

7. Now take two extra deep breaths and then just let your mind float. It is important now to let your mind go to a neutral place. You can just let your mind drift or take yourself to a

beautiful and safe place in your mind, maybe a beach or a garden or just somewhere that feels relaxing.

Now start again at step one and continue to repeat the SWISH process. You will find after some time that the pictures change over very easily and very quickly and that you scarcely have any time to see any of the 'moment of doubt' before it is replaced with the 'perfect birth'. This might be achieved very quickly in as few as five or six ‘swishes’ or may need to be repeated more often until the images change instantly right from the start and without too much thought or effort, or you might find that you simply cannot produce the ‘moment of doubt’ picture at all.

When that happens, you will have changed the negative thought to be positive. Don’t be put off trying this exercise if it sounds a bit complicated. After a few goes you will be surprised just how easy and powerful it can be.

Chapter Sixteen

More techniques for relaxation

Eye Fixation

Remember the brylcreemed doctor in his pin striped suit swinging his pocket watch and commanding 'You are now feeling veeeery sleepy.' You may have wondered what significance the pocket watch held or even why some hypnotists use a black and white swirly spinning wheel to 'hypnotise' their subjects.

Actually the principles behind these are very simple. If you fix your gaze or stare at a fixed point and really focus on it, it becomes easy to focus your mind also. The conscious mind can slow down and clear very quickly and it can act as a short cut to deep relaxation or a quick and easy way of opening up the subconscious.

Read through this exercise and then try it for yourself to see how easy and effective eye fixation can be. If it helps get someone else to read through the steps for you as you try it.

1. Make yourself comfortable, sitting is best.

2. Take a couple of extra deep breaths, breathing all the way in and all the way out.

3. Now find a spot on which to focus your gaze. It's best if the spot is higher up, for example on the ceiling or high up on a wall.

4. Next really stare and focus on that spot and at the same time think about your breath, making sure you are still breathing

fully. Keep staring at the spot almost as if you could look right through it and beyond.

Spend a few minutes totally focusing right on that spot and notice how your mind can also begin to focus and feel more peaceful and how relaxed you can feel. You may even begin to notice how objects in your peripheral vision seem to 'disappear' which is a sign that this is really working for you.

After a few minutes give yourself permission to stop staring or focusing, take another deep breath, have a stretch and remind yourself of where you are and what day and time it is. You may notice the benefits of switching off for a few moments and even be pleasantly surprised at how relaxed and energised you feel afterwards.

This is a useful technique to use for practising relaxation and also to remain focused during birthing. It can be used by both the BW and the BP. It can be used on it's own as a stand alone technique for self hypnosis or as part of another technique. For, example, some hypnobirthing couples will use Eye Fixation as they begin to listen to a hypnobirthing track or as the BP begins to read a script as it can be a good way to 'fast track' to deep relaxation.

Revivification

Take a few moments to remember something that happened in the past that really made you laugh. It doesn't matter what is was or how long ago it was as long as it's something that really tickled your ribs and made you laugh out loud. You might find it helpful to close your eyes for a moment and picture or imagine the scene or hear the words that were spoken.

As you remember that time it is highly likely that you found yourself smiling or even laughing at the thought. It's completely natural when we remember a situation, scenario or conversation that we remember the emotions and feelings connected to that memory. Of course this can work in a negative way and we can remember anxious or sad feelings too but here we are looking to use this natural process for the benefit of the BW and her baby.

By remembering something with positive associations we can summon up or remember the positive feelings attached to that time.

Read through this exercise and then try it for yourself to see how easy and effective revivification can be. If it helps get someone else to read through the steps for you as you try it.

1. Make yourself comfortable, sitting is best.

2. Take a couple of extra deep breaths, breathing all the way in and all the way out.

3. Close your eyes for a moment and take yourself back to a time where you felt very calm and peaceful and your body felt particularly comfortable. It doesn't have to necessarily be anything spectacular, don't think it has to be lying on the beach in Hawaii - it might simply be that feeling of getting into a nice warm and comfortable bed. Just a time when you genuinely felt calm and comfortable.

Spend a few moments really remembering that time and how it felt and as you do take a few extra deep refreshing breaths, breathe in those feelings.

After a few minutes give yourself permission to finish and move back to the present, take another deep breath, have a stretch and remind yourself of where you are and what day and time it is. You may notice how those feelings of calmness and comfort for some time even after you have finished.

Your Beautiful Place

Most people have had the experience of anxiously waiting for news. Maybe waiting for a phone call with news of whether you got a job or an exam result. As you sit and wait time seems to slow down and thoughts buzz around your head, the what ifs and maybes. There's nothing you can do to influence matters, all you can do is wait. Wouldn't it be marvelous if, in situations like that you could be somewhere else altogether. Somewhere very beautiful, peaceful and extremely relaxing. And when you're in this perfect paradise you only think positive thoughts. The exam result or whatever it is becomes unimportant and time really doesn't matter. It could be 10 minutes or 10 hours who cares?! In this beautiful, tranquil haven, time is irrelevant and as you rest there you can just lose track of time. This place is just yours and just for you, it's totally safe, totally secure and totally calm. Like the sound of this place? Like to go there? Well it's easy, because it's right inside your head, right now and you can go there anytime you like, wherever you are and for as long as you want, just by using your imagination.

We all have the ability to daydream or drift off to another place in our mind and this can be extremely helpful if you want to move away from your current situation and change the way you are feeling.

For women during birth it can be part of letting go and letting the birthing body 'get on with things'. Some women find being very present in the birth is important, acknowledging that their body will birth without the need for conscious control, but being very much a part of the birthing. For others it's useful to be somewhere else altogether. Still knowing and understanding that their body knows what to do, allowing that to happen and at the same time remaining calm and relaxed by going to a very lovely place in their mind. One hypnobirthing woman who used this technique throughout most of her hypnobirth said to me, 'I said to the birthing bit of my body "You're ok, you know what to do, you don't need me, you can just get on with it" and I went off to my secret garden and rested there until I was needed again.'

Beautiful Place Exercise

1. Make yourself comfortable, sitting is best.

2. Take a couple of extra deep breaths, breathing all the way in and all the way out.

3. Close your eyes for a moment and imagine yourself at the top of a very beautiful staircase with 10 steps. The staircase can be whatever you want it to be. It might be inside or outside or just somewhere in your imagination, perhaps a lovely wooden staircase leading to a garden with ivy and flowers all around and the starry night sky above you. Remember you're moving down your staircase to a very beautiful place, your favourite place, a very safe and secure place. Perhaps this is a favourite place of yours or simply just somewhere in your imagination. Maybe a beach or a garden or somewhere else all together. Perhaps you're alone or with someone special but here you can be alone and never feel lonely. This is a place where you can be yourself and feel happy, where there's no tension or negative thoughts. A beautiful, tranquil haven. And you can rest as long as you like here in your beautiful place, a day, a week, a month, a year...in hypnosis time, time takes on a new meaning...it's like losing track of time...where 10 minutes can seem like an hour or an hour like ten minutes...so you can come to you

special place wherever and whenever you wish, just by using your imagination.

4. After a while, when you are ready allow yourself to become more aware of your present environment again. You may want to climb back up the staircase up towards your conscious mind or simply open your eyes and become fully aware of where you are and the day and time so you become fully orientated once more.

This technique also has the benefit of time distortion which can be extremely beneficial for the BW. When we relax deeply, the conscious mind relaxes and becomes less active, the subconscious mind opens up and thoughts are unlimited by time and space. The subconscious mind does not have a perception of time. When we sleep the conscious mind rests and the subconscious takes over and creates our dreams. When we wake we may look at the clock to see the time but we do not have a real sense of it. Most of us will have had the experience of feeling like we have just dropped off for five minutes only to wake and find out we've been asleep for much longer. Time distortion can mean it feels like time speeds up or slows down but fundamentally it is losing track of time.

For women who are birthing time distortion is superbly advantageous. It does not matter if birth has taken 2 hours, 6 hours or 15 hours. When a woman begins her birthing she must forget about time altogether. She should remove her watch and turn the clocks around. She must have that trust that her body will let her know when it is time to birth, she must listen to her body and not watch the clock. Midwives and doctors use time as a measure and guide to help them assess how a birth is going. Measuring the dilatation of the cervix by vaginal examination every four hours helps to measure the progress of the birth. Prolonged birth has been shown to be detrimental to both mother and baby and guidelines for practice from bodies such as the National Institute for Clinical Excellence and the World Health Organisation will frequently refer to time limits for birth. This can mean there is an emphasis on time in childbirth. How long has it been? How long it too long? How much longer? How long before we intervene?

Midwives and doctors are dutifully and professionally bound to keep an eye on the time and the rate of a birth they attend. The BW must, therefore, hand over the time keeping to the midwife. She should consider asking the midwife and the birthing partner not to refer to time. Her birthing body will tell her when it's time and if she is peaceful and calm it really will not matter to her how long it takes.

Turning up the dial exercise

What a wonderful, phenomenal, extraordinary thing the imagination is! It can help us to feel good, relaxed and confident, it can take us to exotic places, it can prepare us for almost anything. Using the imagination to 'pretend', rehearse or prepare can be one of our most powerful inner resources and with practice we can use it to overcome fear, build confidence as well as to instantly and deeply relax, the benefits of using our imagination as a tool are far reaching. The good news is that we all have an imagination and all have the ability to use it for our benefit. Children use their imagination all the time and with ease, creating stories and games with endless fantastical possibilities. Some adults feel they lose their imagination as they get older but this simply is not the case. Think of the imagination as a muscle, the more you use it and exercise it the stronger it gets and the easier it is to use. As we mature the stresses and strains of adulthood and responsibility can swamp the conscious mind and the imagination becomes neglected and weak. By working and exercising the imagination though we can get it up and running and working for our benefit.

Using your imagination to 'Turn up the Dial' on positive feelings is a simple yet powerful way to increase and intensify those feelings and feel really good.

Turning up the Dial Exercise

1. Read through this exercise and then try it for yourself to see how easy and effective it can be. If it helps get someone else to read through the steps for you as you try it.

2. Make yourself comfortable, sitting is best.

3. Take a couple of extra deep breaths, breathing all the way in and all the way out.

4. Close your eyes for a moment and take yourself back to a time where you felt very calm and very confident. It doesn't have to necessarily be anything amazing, don't think it has to be winning the London Marathon - it might simply be that you met a deadline or had a great chat with a friend. It's fine too if it was only for a few moments, just remember how it felt.

5. Now in your mind's eye imagine a large dial, it can be any design and colour you want it to be and it has the numbers 1 all the way up to 10 on it. At the moment the dial is at 1 but after a couple of extra deep refreshing breaths you are going to very gently and very easily turn that dial up. As you do allow those feelings of calm confidence to increase with every number. Let the dial move up and up 2...3...4.. all the way up to 10. As you reach 10 feel those feelings of calm confidence have completely filled your entire being so you are completely filled with calm confidence.

6. After a while, when you are ready allow yourself to become more aware of your present environment again. Leave your dial up at 10 and bring back that calm confidence with you, open your eyes and become fully aware of where you are and the day and time so you become fully orientated once more.

Chapter Seventeen

Home birth/Waterbirth/Hypnobirth

At 2am one October morning I was called out to a home birth. I remember clearly it was a Saturday night and the clocks had just gone back. It was freezing cold and the rain lashed down as I drove somewhat wearily to the address. I hadn't met this family before and their home wasn't on my normal patch so, as I made my way down the Old Kent Road I began to feel the tension of uncertainty, wondering what lay ahead for me that night. The sat nav did it's thing and I found the address easily, it was a flat in a gated community without parking. I circled the block a couple of times, the tension rising as all I could see before me was a seemingly endless stream of double red or yellow lines (despite what many people think community midwives cannot park anywhere!). All this time I expected my phone to ring with an angry birthing partner at the other end wondering where on earth I was but thankfully it didn't. I finally found a spot to park which was about a 10 minute walk to the flat and so I hurriedly dragged my bags out of the boot and blustered my way towards my destination. I stood at the tall ominous gates which were the entrance to the flats. Shivering, I rung the bell. I could feel a headache coming on, was very cold and tired and now wasn't even sure whether it was 2am or 3am, had I put my watch back...er forward..oh what time *is* it really! No-one seemed to be answering the bell, so I decided to call the number I had for the birthing partner. No answer. I paused for a moment, this really wasn't my idea of fulfilling midwifery, maybe I was in the wrong job. Finally a rather drunk man in a slightly disheveled business suit staggered along, swayed for a moment in front of the gate and then beeped himself through. I quickly followed him in. Now all I had to do was figure out the bizarre and nonsensical numbering system of the flats and I was there. It started to rain again. Feeling like I was participating in a NHS version of the Crystal Maze I wandered aimlessly until almost by accident I spotted the correct flat and I noticed the door had been left ajar. So cold, wet, tired, miserable and despondent I bundled my way through the door and the scene I came upon as I did so nearly made me weep tears of joy! The flickering candles gave light to Maisy as she serenely floated in the birthing pool. She was sitting very upright in the water with her arms resting on the edge of the pool, her long wet hair rested perfectly on her shoulders. It struck me how beautiful she looked - women birthing in water often look quite goddess like, I think. As I stood in the doorway I began to feel my shoulders relaxing, this was going to be good, I could feel it. Her partner, Cliff, was right next to Maisy sitting on the floor on the outside of the pool. He turned to me and smiled, he looked totally chilled. I became aware that my headache seemed so much easier now and I was really not concerned whether it was 2am or 3am, all was fine here. Soft music played in the background and wafts of lavender floated through the air. I too sat down by the edge of the pool, took a deep breath and remembered why I loved being a midwife so much. This was perfect, Maisy didn't want or need anything, to all intents and purposes she looked like she was sleeping. Occasionally she opened her eyes and asked for a drink but soon she would close her eyes again as she continued to float. After a short while of being there it struck me that the calmness and peace at this birth had a familiarity. I asked Maisy's partner if they were hypnobirthing. 'Of course.' came the answer.

Around 2 hours after my arrival Maisy birthed very easily and gently, her little girl peacefully floated up out of the water to meet her and nuzzled her breast almost immediately.

Maisy had had an induction with her first baby two years earlier and had felt very out of control right from the beginning. With this, her second birth, she had been determined to do everything within her power to stay in control and after discovering hypnobirthing realised that learning to be calm and confident would bring with it the composure she needed. For Maisy too being at home was important so she could feel relaxed and in control. For many BW being in their own home means they feel safe and secure in familiar surroundings. Being able to drink tea from their favorite mug, sit on their own loo or snuggle on their own pillows helps. Also if you are birthing in your own home anyone who arrives is a visitor on your territory. The midwife is your guest rather than you their patient. He/she is there only for you and your baby's needs rather than you being told where to go and what to do and expected to comply with the rules and regulations of the hospital setting. Women who opt to birth at home will often say that one of the main reasons they choose to do so is because they know they will feel more relaxed at home rather than in hospital.

At Maisy's birthing the combination of hypno/home and waterbirth were marvelous. Hypnobirthing women frequently prefer to birth in water as they go so well together. Almost without exception women getting into a birthing pool will give a long sigh of relief and their whole body visibly relaxes. Once in the pool most women will opt to stay in and birth in the water, even those who may not have been too sure whether they would like it. The benefits of birthing in water are widely documented (Cluet and Burns 2009) and it is not my intention to go into too much detail here but just to say that the warmth and buoyancy of the water are great for the BW to feel relaxed and comfortable as well as for making the transition into the world for the baby so very subtle and gentle. When a baby moves from the warm watery sac in the womb to the warm watery birth pool then straight to the warm skin of mummy there is little to stimulate them to complain or cry and so it's no surprise that hypno and water babies are noticeably calmer at birth.

For more information, including a jargon free, comprehensive look at evidence and research visit www.homebirth.co.uk

Chapter Eighteen

Practice

All of the techniques mentioned should be practised by the hypnobirthing couple as often as possible. They may find that one particular technique works really well for them and so they focus on being relaxed and confident using just one or two techniques. Others will find it best to practise all of the techniques so that they have them all at their disposal during the birth should they feel they need them. Practice is key and for the greater majority of people it is needed so that at the time of the birth the techniques become second nature, easy to use and thus more effective.

Tips for Practising

1. Make hypnobirthing part of your life. Do some practising every day. Make hypnobirthing part of who you are, embrace the ideas and absorb the philosophy. This way when the time for birthing comes it will all happen quite naturally and without effort.

2. Visualise. Take any opportunity to have a mental rehearsal for the birth. Imagine yourself feeling great, looking good and everything going perfectly. If you were going for a job interview or performing in a show you would rehearse beforehand so why not for birth? Sitting on the bus or waiting for your antenatal appointment just close your eyes take a deep breath and daydream.

3. Practise anytime, anywhere. You don't need to be tucked up in bed with total silence to be in a deeply relaxed state. Deep relaxation means the body is free of tension and the mind is at peace, this state is possible anywhere. Even if you were standing, walking or in a place with noise and bright

lights it is possible to feel serene, tranquil and totally relaxed. Most women given the space to do what comes naturally during birth will stand and walk so it's important to know you can still be totally relaxed even when being upright and moving around. Consider practising whilst sitting or kneeling or maybe leaning over a birthing ball or sitting back to front on a chair. These are all good positions for birthing. Many hypnobirthing women practise on their commute by train to work in order to make practicing part of their everyday routine (obviously not advisable if commuting by car!). One hypnobirthing mum told me how she listened to her hypnobirthing track every morning on the tube. She reckoned that if she could feel calm and relaxed at 8am on on the London Underground, when no-one had given her a seat then she could feel calm and relaxed anywhere! She did indeed go on to have her baby at home in water in just 4 hours, lovely!

4. Practise together. The hypnobirthing techniques are as much for the birthing partner as they are for the mother. It is important that the BP feels calm and relaxed for their own sake, so they too have a good experience when meeting their baby. Also it is incredibly helpful for the BW if she has a peaceful, calm companion. One hypnobirthing dad took a hypnobirthing track with him on a long haul flight. Normally quite a nervous passenger he was amazed at how relaxed he was and how quickly time passed. He laughed as he told me it really didn't matter to him that the track mentioned 'your birthing body' or 'your perineum'. Even though the hypnobirthing track was intended for pregnant women it still guided his breathing and subconscious mind into a deeply relaxed place.

5. Breathe! The resounding message that is heard over and over in hypnobirthing stories is how important good breathing is. 'It was all in the breathing' or 'I couldn't have done it without the breathing' are heard again and again. The benefits of breathing fully have already been discussed but it's important to reiterate the need for practice.

Chapter Nineteen

Optimal Fetal Positioning

Much has been written about Optimal Fetal Positioning (OFP) in recent years and it is not my intention to try to replicate the in depth and significant work of Jean Sutton and Pauline Scott (www.homebirth.org 2012). However as the position of the baby during a birth is so important I feel the need to at least outline the principles. I would urge anyone who hasn't already visited www.homebirth.org to do so as in my opinion this information should be given as a priority to pregnant women.

Jean Sutton is a midwife and Pauline Scott an antenatal teacher. Together they developed the theory that a pregnant woman could influence the position of her baby by being conscious of their movement and posture. Many difficult births and numerous interventions are as a result of the unborn baby being in the wrong position so it becomes difficult or even impossible for them to move through the pelvis to be born. By encouraging her baby into a good position for birth the pregnant woman can make her birth quicker and easier.

Ideally the unborn baby should lie with their head downwards towards the bottom of the womb (and by 36 weeks 97% of babies do) the baby's back should also be towards the front of Mum's tummy. The baby should be nicely curled up in a ball with their chin on their chest. In this position they don't have far to go to be born, with just a quarter of a turn they will very easily move down and fit through the pelvis. This position is often referred to as Occiput Anterior or O.A. which simply means the back of the baby's head (Occiput) towards the front (Anterior) of the mother's pelvis. It is essential that the baby has their chin on their chest so that the smallest diameter of the head is coming first which means they will fit through the pelvis easily. If they have their chin up a wider part comes first and it can be more difficult.

If the baby is head down but with it's back towards the mother's back (often called back to back or spine to spine) it would be described as Occiput Posterior or O.P. which simply means the back of the baby's head towards the back of the pelvis.

The O.P. position also means the smallest diameter of the baby's head is not coming first and it can be associated with a long and painful labour. Occasionally some babies will fit through the pelvis in the O.P. position but this is unusual. Most babies need to turn all the way round around into the O.A position first before they can move downwards and this can take a long time, often days of birthing. Sometimes babies in the O.P. positions don't turn or move down into the pelvis at all and get wedged in the pelvis and need to be born by caesarean section.

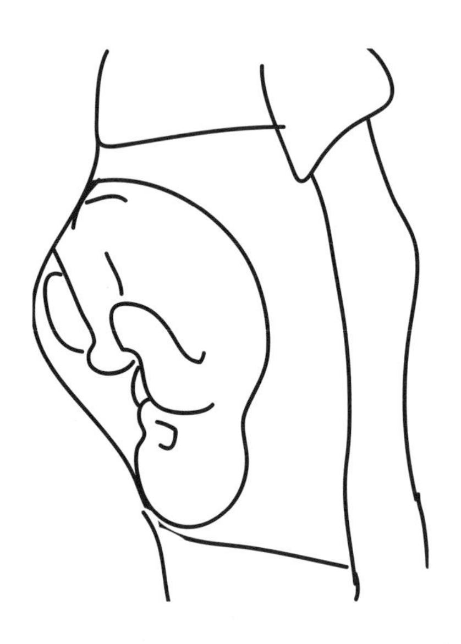

Occiput Posterior

Most babies in the O.A. position will lie with their back towards the left side of their mum, this is called Left Occiput Anterior or L.O.A. (see diagram below) and it is said that babies who lie with their back towards to the right of mum's tummy (Right Occiput Anterior, R.O.A.)

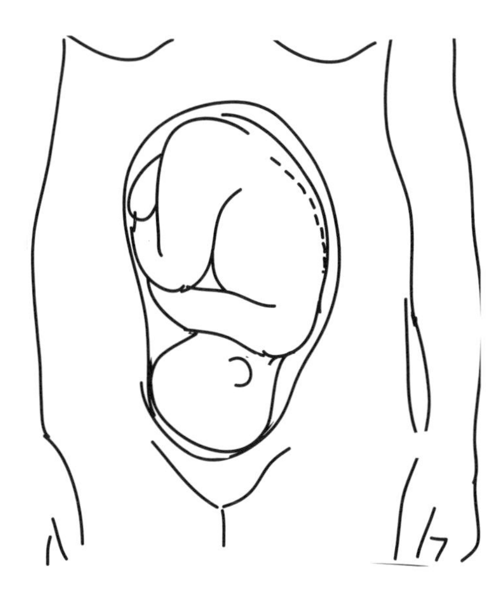
Left Occiput Anterior

are more likely to turn around into an O.P. position. Generally speaking babies tend to turn clockwise with the muscular tightenings of surges during birth and so a baby who is R.O.A may turn around to be O.P. before it turns to be L.O.A. This is a generalisation, however, and midwives will report a good number of births where babies are R.O.A. before birth and remain so during birth as well.

The good news is that the pregnant woman can influence and encourage their babies to turn into a good position for birth and below is an outline of what can be done.

Relaxation

It stands to reason that when a pregnant woman relaxes deeply she gives her baby her the space they need to move. As she physically relaxes she will relax her abdominal muscles and her pelvic floor muscles giving the baby more room for manoeuvre. Deep breathing will send optimum levels of oxygen to the baby giving them the energy they need to move as well. I firmly believe that the unborn baby instinctively wants to get into an O.A. position. Most fetus will end up head down in the womb (we don't really know how this happens, it seems to be an instinctive reflex) surely then, it stands to reason that the fetus will also reflexively get into the best position to fit through the pelvis and be born - it just needs to be given the space to do so. Chronic tension that often results from modern living will mean the abdominal muscles and pelvic floor muscles don't relax deeply enough or often enough to give the baby space to move. Practising hypnobirthing techniques, deep breathing, yoga or just taking time out to really relax will mean the baby has every opportunity to turn to where they want to be in the O.A. position.

Activity

A modern sedentary lifestyle often means we are not as active as we should be. In the case of the pregnant woman it will also mean that the pelvis doesn't move enough or in the right way so as to encourage the baby to move in a downwards spiral so as to engage in the pelvis.

The pregnant woman can encourage the baby to move into the O.A. position by being upright, keeping the pelvis open and moving it in the correct way.

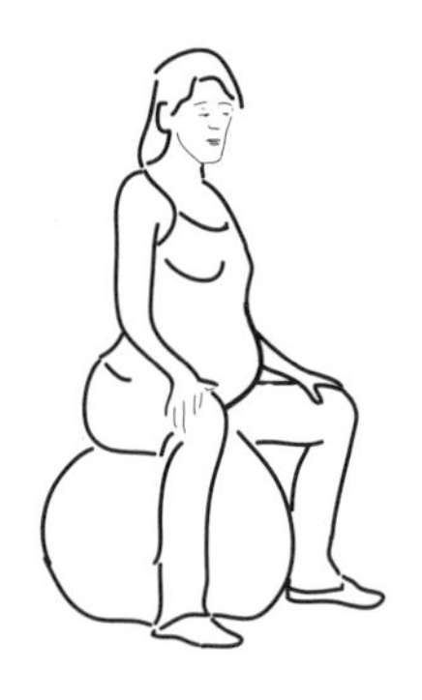

The baby's back is the heaviest side of its body. This means that its back will naturally move or swing towards which ever side of the tummy or abdomen (or bump) is lowest. If the front or outermost part of the pregnant tummy is lowest, for example whilst sitting back to front on a chair leaning forward, then the baby's back will tend to swing towards the front of the tummy into an O.A. position. If the back is lower than the bump, e.g. whilst lying back or leaning back on a deep seated sofa, then the baby's back is more likely swing towards the mother's back.

When sitting the pregnant woman should sit with her knees apart and her feet flat on the floor, again it's best if the knees are lower than the hips. She should then lean forwards slightly so her back is at an angle and her pelvis tilted slightly.

Activities such as swimming, walking and pilates will bring about a gentle and fluid movement of the pelvis which will encourage the baby to turn.

Hands and Knees Position

It is thought that a hands and knees position which puts the pelvis higher than the head is useful for turning a baby into L.O.A. position. This position (see diagram) means that the front of mum's tummy is right down and, therefore, the heaviest part of the baby (the back) will swing around towards the front. It may be helpful to think that as the pregnant tummy is down it acts almost like a hammock for the baby. Many pregnant women find this position surprisingly comfortable as it stretches out the back and pelvis muscles. It may also be helpful to crawl whilst in this position in order to encourage the joints of the pelvis to

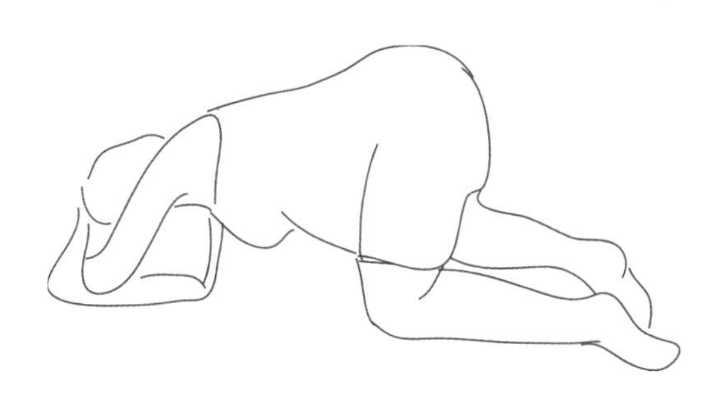

move. Although it can be a peculiar sight to see a heavily pregnant woman on her hands and knees with her bottom in the air crawling around it does seem to work.

Very early one Summer's morning I arrived at the home of Dana and Harvey. Dana, who was planning to birth in hospital, was in the earlier part of her birthing. The midwifery team I worked with at the time had the luxury of being able to visit all their birthing women at their home to begin with. This meant that women could choose during the birthing itself whether to stay at home or move to hospital and because of this many women, even those planning a hospital birth, would opt to stay and birth in the comfort and familiar surroundings of their own home. As I made my way to Dana and Harvey's house I quietly wished to myself that this couple had prepared for their birth using hypnobirthing as both were tense and anxious, which I knew could only be unhelpful. I had been on call the previous night and Harvey had called me twice to say that although the surges were irregular and mild both he and Dana were concerned that it had been like that for around 48hrs. My initial assessment was that everything was fine and there was nothing to worry about but with the second phone call I decided that they might benefit from some TLC and a face to face chat to reassure them. On entering the couple's sitting room I was surprised and a little perturbed to see Dana lying on her back on her sofa. I'm not quite sure why she was like that as she was particularly distressed, I can only presume that she thought she was supposed to lie down because it certainly wasn't a good place for her to be. I sat with them both for a while, trying to be a calm presence which was a little challenging as Harvey anxiously chatted at my side about everything and nothing, his anxiety seemed to make words fall from his mouth. After observing Dana for around an hour I noticed that her surges were very short (maybe 30 or 40 seconds in length) and had no pattern or rhythm to them at all. Dana reported that her baby was nicely wriggling around but that she felt she couldn't cope anymore as she felt so tired. So then, with her permission, I had a feel of her baby through her tummy (the correct term for this is an abdominal examination but midwives often refer to it as a palpation) and as I did I wasn't too surprised at what I felt. The baby was completely back to back with Dana (sometimes called a direct O.P.) and all I could feel were little hands, knees and feet poking forwards. I wasn't too surprised with this finding for several reasons. Firstly the shape Dana's bump was a give away, OP babies often have a classic dip at the tummy (see illustration on page 124) and Dana's bump had just this. Secondly I felt that being tense, anxious and lying down might have all contributed to Dana's baby not turning in the way it needed to. The final clue was the hours of short irregular surges which might have been because the baby wasn't descending into the pelvis and, therefore, coming down onto the cervix (the baby descending onto the cervix will release oxytocin and help to move a birthing along).

I told Dana that her baby needed to turn and suggested the best way to do that would be for her to change position. When I mentioned a hands and knees position she almost leaped into the air and flipped over onto all fours. It was like she was relieved at being given permission to move. Dana seemed instantly more in control and more comfortable in this position. Now with each surge instead of crying out for help she gave out a deep low hum with each out breath and instinctively swayed her hips from side to side. She stayed like this for some time, her bottom stuck up in the air and her face nuzzled into a soft velvet cushion on her sofa. As Harvey watched all this he had become much quieter and although I think he wasn't too sure what was going on he was more reassured as Dana was so much less distressed now. Over the next 3 or 4 hours Dana interspersed a hands and knees position with walking. Every so often she would rise up from her red velvet cushion, stretch and take some time to walk around the room, then after a while she would sink back to all fours. It was around 8am and I noticed the day was already warm, I noticed too that Dana's surges where much more regular and stronger now. A surge would arrive around every 3 minutes and last for a minute or more. The baby's heartbeat and movements were good and a quick feel of the Dana's bump revealed that she had turned all the way around to L.O.A. In just a few hours of moving instinctively and in the right way Dana had turned her baby into a good position for birth. My shift was finishing and I handed over to the morning midwife with a real sense of satisfaction. Dana's baby had literally turned a corner and her birthing had done so too. It was even more satisfying to hear later that afternoon that Dana had opted to stay at home and had birthed her baby around lunchtime, just a few hours after I left.

Chapter Twenty

Massage

Massage is extremely popular with birthing women. I have lost count of the number of births I have attended where massage was not just a part of the support mechanism for the BW but an integral part of it.

Massage is very relaxing and supportive. It will increase the circulation as well as encourage the release of endorphins and oxytocin. For many women the physical, supportive touch of their BP through massage is essential for them to remain relaxed and calm throughout birth.

Research into massage during childbirth has been shown to ease pain and reduce anxiety (NCCWCH 2007: 94-5; Chang et al 2006; Chang et al 2002). It is also linked with quicker births and a lower risk of postnatal depression. (Simkin et al 2004).

Below is described a massage technique that has been developed for BP to learn. It incorporates deep breathing, anchors and hormone releasing touch. The massage is best done straight onto the skin with a massage oil such as sweet almond or grapeseed oil.

1. Firstly the BW must be comfortable. For practicing I suggest she sits back to front on a chair with a pillow on the back of the chair. Please note if the BW chooses to sit on a birthing ball then make sure there is something in front of her to lean on for support and stability (a chair, table or window ledge, for example).

2. Next the BP needs to be comfortable also. The BP needs to be behind the BW and lower down. It is important for the

BP to keep their hips and shoulders square and not to twist the spine.

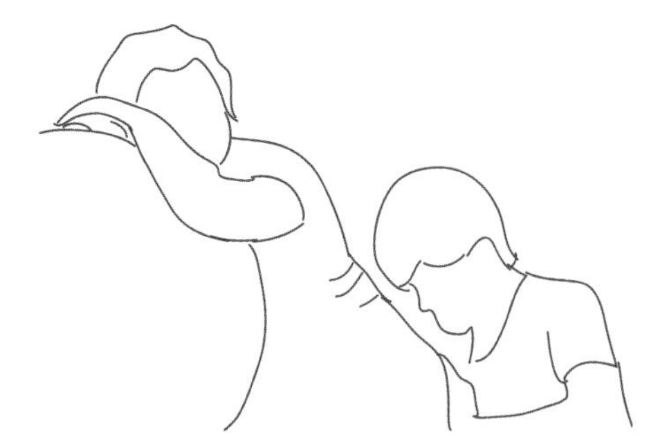

3. The BP places their hands on the lower back. The hands should be very relaxed and resting flat against the back.

4. The BP then moves their hands smoothly up towards the shoulders being careful to keep their hands at either side of, and away from, the spine in the centre of the back.

5. At the same time the BW breathes all the way in so that the up stroke of the massage coincides with the deep inhalation.

6. As the BW then breathes out slowly the BP places their hands on the BWs shoulders and applies very gentle downwards pressure.

7. During the next breath the BP will move their hands down the body towards the base of the back ready to start this again. As they move their hands downwards they should very very lightly drum or tap using the ends of the fingers across the back (this light touch will encourage the release of endorphins and oxytocin). If drumming fingers are too tickly then as an alternative the BP can make 'S' shaped, stroking movements with the ends of the fingers as they move

downwards. At the end of this breath the hands should be ready again at the base of the back to repeat from step 1.

As with all other techniques this massage technique should be practised. Every couple is different and many adapt this technique to suit them. Some find a light stroking touch useful, others prefer pressure on the deeper tissues. During practice couples can explore what works for them and the BP can feel relaxed knowing what the BW is likely to find helpful.

Tip: To help the BP coincide the massage stroke with the breath the BW should make the breath audible, breathing in and out deeply and letting the air moving in and out to make a noise will guide the BP and also encourage deep breathing.

It is important to mention that not all birthing women will want massage, for some BW it is important not to be touched and they may feel they need to be given space to focus on breathing and relaxation. For those women it is almost like they are in a bubble, anyone being too near the bubble might burst it and disturb them, they will want to know loving support is near by but not too near.

Chapter Twenty One

Birth Preferences

Someone once said that a good birth plan can be written on a post-it note. I presume this tongue in cheek comment suggests it's best not to plan too much. As a midwife I have come across birth plans that are so detailed they take up 3 or 4 sides of A4 or ones that have been burned to CD and distributed to anyone who might be interested. I often feel that these kind of ultra-detailed and specific birth plans are a woman's (or couple's) attempt to retain some control on a situation in which they are feeling out of control of. They are trying to control their circumstances, where they will birth, how they will birth etc. by detailing every possible twist or turn their birth may take. Of course every BW and her partner will have a way they would prefer things to go. Perhaps preferring to birth in water, to be able to move around freely, maybe for the BP to cut the umbilical cord or to receive the baby. It is important though to see these as preferences and not a definite plan. A birth plan that doesn't go to plan might be seen as a failed plan. There is no failure in birthing, it is a phenomenal and magical process through which women and their partners get to meet their babies. Calmness and relaxation will encourage that process to go smoothly but even if it doesn't entirely go the way you would prefer it doesn't have to be a negative, scary or out of control experience. The real magic of hypnobirthing is that it teaches BW to use their own internal resources to feel good and stay calm and that peace can be transported anywhere. A hypnobirthing couple who were planning a home birth/ waterbirth/hypnobirth ended up with an emergency caesarean section (a decision they were happy with and made along with their obstetrician), as their baby had become distressed towards the end of the birthing. As the mother described the moment she was whisked into theatre she spoke of the importance of knowing that she needed to continue to breathe deeply and all the way through the operation she remained calm and in control. One remark she made has always stuck with me, she said, 'You know, even though it was the opposite kind of birth than the one we were planning, I still enjoyed the birth of my baby!' This couple met their baby boy with calmness and after being yanked unceremoniously into the world it must have been lovely to settle on the calm, smiling chest of his mummy.

So although BW and their BPs will have preferences for their birth they should remember that ultimately they cannot control their circumstances fully. What they do have control over is how they feel and how they react, their internal resources will give them control over themselves, the ultimate control.

Five Steps to Writing Birthing Preferences

1. Keep it succinct and simple. Think and talk in generic terms, avoid being too specific. About 7 or 8 bullet points should do it (see sample below).

2. Be flexible and open minded, use phrases such as 'we prefer' or 'ideally we would like'.

3. Write in a chronological way. Start with what you would prefer during the early and active phases of birth, then when the baby is born then moving on to the cutting of the cord and placenta then breastfeeding etc.

4. Make the preferences personal to you. Avoid the temptation to cut and paste someone else's birthing preferences. This is about you and what you prefer.

5. Rather than a long list of 'I don't want..' and 'I do want..' consider asking to avoid any unnecessary intervention and

disruption and if anything is recommended to be fully informed and consented beforehand. All those requests such as 'I don't want to be induced' or 'I don't want an episiotomy' or 'I want to be free to move around' are covered in this statement.

6. If possible show your birthing preferences to your midwife either at an antenatal appointment or when you meet them during your birthing. Most maternity units provide space in the notes for you to write you preferences or provide a tick box list. Make sure you keep a copy of your preferences for yourself as well.

Below is a sample of the kind of birthing preferences you might put together.

Sample Birth Preferences

*We are looking forward to a gentle, calm birth and to this end have been practising various hypnobirthing relaxation and positive conditioning techniques. We respect your role and responsibility as an attending birth professional and thank you for your support as we look forward to meeting our baby.

*We would like to keep our birth as 'normal' as possible and avoid any unnecessary intervention. Should any intervention be recommended we would like to be fully informed and consented beforehand.

*I would like to use the birthing pool/shower/bath to help me to relax during birth.

*I would like to be given the space to move around and whatever way I need to so I can follow my instincts during birth.

*I would like to continue to breathe deeply during the second stage and birth of my baby and not be directed to push or not to push.

*Please allow the cord to stop pulsating before it is cut by (name).

*Please allow the afterbirth to be delivered naturally.

*Please put baby skin to skin immediately at birth (either with mummy or daddy) and only break skin to skin if absolutely necessary and with our consent. Please provide assistance to encourage early breastfeeding.

*We consent/do not consent to Vitamin K by injection/orally.

Chapter Twenty Two

Birthing Positions

If a BW is given the mental, emotional and physical space to do what comes naturally she will almost always move in such a way that will be conducive to birth her baby without complication. Most women choose to walk, kneel or stand and will instinctively sway or squat during a surge.

Antenatal classes will traditionally 'teach' good positions for the mother for birth and many will ask couples attending to practise the positions together. Although I agree that there is some benefit to this I do not think it is absolutely necessary. For some women moving into good positions for birth can act as a mental rehearsal and give them permission, if you like, that it is acceptable to get onto all fours or squat and more importantly for them to know that it is not helpful to lie on their back.

Lying on your back when pregnant and birthing is uncomfortable and can be detrimental to birth. It will mean that the sacrum (the triangular bone at the base of the back) and the coccyx (the tail bone) will be pushed inwards and the space in the pelvis through which the baby needs to pass will become smaller. It also means the angle of the pelvis will be wrong and the baby will be trying to move 'uphill' wasting energy whilst fighting gravity.

As a student midwife I learnt all of the above and so understood the need to be upright to allow gravity to help the downwards journey for the baby as well as the importance of allowing the pelvis to be as open as possible. As I moved through my training I found it perplexing, therefore, why some women would almost seem stuck to the bed and how, even with encouragement would find it almost impossible to move. As a newly qualified midwife I remember being with a woman who had agreed to be induced because she had become overdue. With her permission I had broken her waters and now I knew how important it was for her to get up and move around. As I suggested this to her she gave me a look of astonishment mixed with horror. 'But I can't get up!' she exclaimed. For a moment I hesitate, maybe I had made an awful faux pas and had missed something, maybe she has a physical disability and I had been totally insensitive. 'Why can't you get up?' I replied gingerly. With wide eyes she replied, 'Because I'm having a baby!' So I took some time to explain the benefits to her and her baby of getting off the bed, being upright and moving around. She listened intently and when I had finished she paused for a second, shook her head and said, 'No, I'm not having a home birth you know, I'm in hospital, anyway I've seen it on the TV you've got to lie down, otherwise what's this bed for!'

The physical environment as well as birthing professional's attitudes can profoundly affect the position women may choose for birth (Albers 2007). Birthing professionals may, even on a subconscious level, prefer a woman to lie down. From their point of view it might feel easier to see the birth and the it may feel more contained, even safer. The reality is that lying down can ultimately make birth more difficult even less safe and it has now become widely accepted that moving around freely during birth (active birthing) is preferable (Royal College of Midwives 2005).

So practising birthing positions may be helpful by giving women permission to move in this way as well as empower ing them with the knowledge of the best way to move during birth.

If a BW understands and trusts her birthing body, if she truly believes that she can birth, if she trusts and understands that it she doesn't need to make any conscious effort and that it will happen all by itself then I am convinced she will move in the right way.

Standing and Walking

Many BW will instinctively walk during birth and often find they intuitively like to stand and lean forwards, perhaps supported by their partner or leaning onto a stair banister or window ledge. Walking creates a beautifully gentle and fluid movement of the pelvis and leaning forward will mean the pelvis is at a slight angle. Having the pelvis tilted in this way is thought to increase the inlet of the pelvis and line the baby up at the best angle to move into it. It is possible it also encourages the baby to put their chin on their chest which helps them to move downwards through the pelvis.

During a surge BW who are following their instincts will often sway or circle the hips. This pelvic movement will also encourage the baby to turn and move lower into the pelvis. A BW who breathes deeply and sways during a surge creates a soothing rhythm which is powerfully hypnotic to watch.

Squatting

Moving down into a semi squat is natural way for birthing women to move. It's common for women to sink down and bend the knees during a surge sometimes as a response to the feelings of heaviness or downwards pressure as the baby moves down. Sitting on the toilet, a birthing stool or a birthing ball will mean a semi squat position is adopted, this opens the pelvis and encourages the downwards path of the baby. Some women will instinctively move into a very deep squat especially during the birthing phase. A deep squat can be very useful to open the pelvis but care must be taken to only go into a squat with the heels still on the floor. It is thought that a squatting position with the heels off the floor may tip the pelvis into an angle where the baby cannot easily move into or turn the pelvis. Some say to avoid deep squatting in late pregnancy or before the baby is fully engaged to avoid the baby moving into the O.P. position. In my experience it seems that some women will intuitively squat and where squatting is done naturally and with ease it will be a good position for birth. For others if squatting is more conscious (some women will squat because they have read or heard that it is a good position for birth) and does not come so naturally it often means that the whole thing is harder work and not so useful. Once again I think that BW should do what feels right and comes naturally and trust that their body will tell them what they need to do to birth their baby.

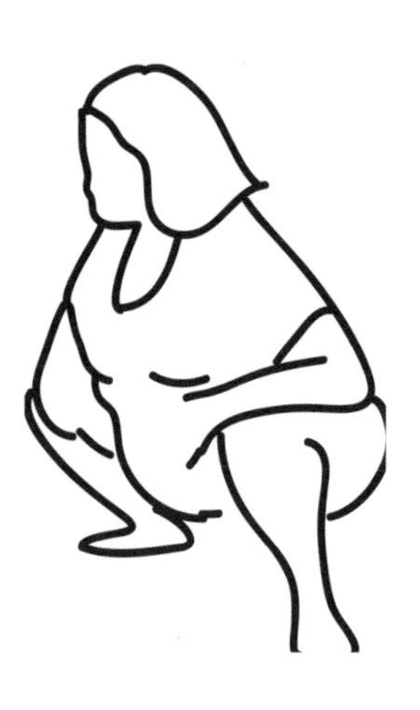

Hands and Knees or Kneeling

Kneeling and all fours positions are possibly one of the most instinctively common positions for birthing and particularly for the actual birth itself. These positions are perfect for birth, they mean the BW remains upright and encourage the pelvis to move and be open. BW will again often sway or circle the hips in whilst on all fours and at the same time they are able to rest and relax the upper body and head. Resting the upper body and head is important for these positions and many women enjoy kneeling on pillows on the floor whilst leaning over their sofa, again made comfortable with lots of pillows and cushions. In hospitals and birth centres women will make use of large bean bags, birthing balls and floor mats to be comfortable on all fours. It's important to protect the knees in these positions and the birthing partner should take care to ensure the BW has a cushion or pillow under each knee. Kneeling and leaning over a birthing ball works well too. The BW can circle the ball around with her arms and upper body and this will move the pelvis very gently, this position is also useful for stretching out and relaxing tense and achy back muscle.

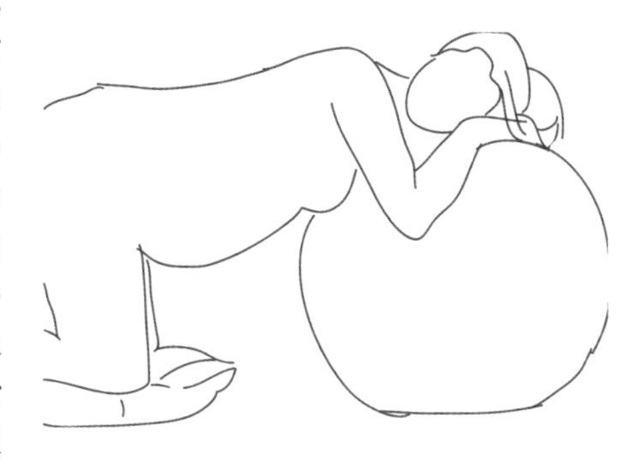

The birthing pool

In the birthing pool the buoyancy of the water often means that the BW is free to float and the BW movement tends to be more fluid. The buoyancy also means that there is much less pressure on the sacrum even in a sitting position. Sitting upright leaning on the edge of the pool is a comfortable place for many women. Again it means she is upright so gravity helps her and by keeping her knees apart and swishing her bottom around in the water will keep the pelvis moving and open.

The mantra for hypnobirthing women with regards to moving during childbirth is 'if it feels good do it!' Sitting for long periods of time is bad for our circulation and joints. Because of this our bodies become uncomfortable and we naturally shift around and move our bodies every so often to remain comfortable and this in turn will move our joints and increase the circulation to the muscles. Generally our bodies instinctively tell us when we need to move for our own wellbeing and childbirth is no exception to this.

Chapter Twenty Three

The Early Phase of Birthing

It is very common for birthing woman to experience a gradual onset to birth, the surges and the sensations associated with them. This gentle, graduate, progressive build up to birth can be very useful, particularly from an emotional point of view. It can mean that birthing women have plenty of time to 'get into the zone' or to get themselves into a deeply relaxed and confident place.

The early phase of birth is sometimes referred to as 'early labour' or the 'latent phase' and is the time it takes for the neck of the womb to soften and thin out, going from it's pre-birth 3-4cm long to being paper thin and opening to around 4cm dilated. During this time the baby is likely to move further down into the pelvis and maybe even turn as it does so. It does vary but for the majority of birthing women this phase of birth is accompanied by mild, irregular surges. The surges will come and go but without any particular pattern or rhythm and tend to be quite short in length.

How the BW and her BP approaches and reacts to this part of the birth can make all the difference to how they are able to manage and carry on to the more active phase of birth.

The two most important things to remember during this part of the birthing are;

1. This is a normal and useful part of birthing and

2. This isn't the birthing time yet, it's the warm up and may take time

Remember Mable in the Introduction? She represents the women I have met over the years who have not been prepared and have not understood the two points above. As soon as she felt some mild, irregular surges she immediately presumed that it was 'labour'. Then she is immediately tense and anxious, she doesn't rest or care for herself and wastes her energy on tense muscles and quick shallow breathing. Also when her baby doesn't arrive soon she presumes that there is something wrong with her birth and her body. For hypnobirthing women it is different. Women who use hypnobirthing for their birth preparation will understand that this earlier phase is important and useful but also that it may take some time. They will understand that their birthing body will know what do to and there is no need to force or resist what is happening. They will know the need for relaxation and rest, they will have techniques to help them to conserve their energy for where it is needed i.e. the birthing bit of their body. So as they enter into the more active part of birth they still have the resources they need to carry on, they are calm, composed and in control.

7 Top Tips for the Early Phase of Birth

1. Let it happen. Trust that your body knows what to do and when to do it. Don't try to control what is happening or the pace. Remember the softening and thinning of the cervix, the surges and the movement of the baby will all happen automatically. There's no need to try, just breathe and relax.

2. There's no rush, forget about time. Time distortion (see page 112) can be so useful during this phase of birth and it's important to remember that it can take time. There is no set time for this phase and it can start and stop too. If you are at all worried about yourself or your baby then you should get checked out by a midwife but if you are well and the baby is moving around then it's most likely that all there is to do is

wait. NB the baby's movements should remain the same during the early phase as during your pregnancy. If there is any change in the baby's movements then speak to your midwife and get a check.

3. Drink! Keep hydrated. The body needs fluid to work well especially when it is working to birth your baby. Drink lots of water and energizing drinks such as fresh fruit juice and fruit smoothies.

4. Eat! Take in easily digestible, high energy foods. Your body needs energy from calories to function well. Taking in fluids and calories will keep your energy levels up.

5. Balance activity with rest. It is important to keep upright and to keep the pelvis open and moving so as to allow the baby to move down and into the pelvis and many women will instinctively want to move and walk during the early phase. Slow gentle walking will be enough and the BW should avoid 'route marching' for hours in order to try and 'get things going' and wearing herself out. It's important to move around but also to conserve energy so that even if this phase takes a while it really doesn't matter. Being deeply relaxed and physically free of tension will mean no energy is wasted.

Tip: To remain upright and still rest during the early phase, rather than lie down, sit back to front on a dining chair. Cover the back of the chair with a thick blanket and a pillow. Rest your head onto the pillow and let your arms hang loosely at your sides.

6. Encourage oxytocin. Deep breathing, relaxation, massage and nipple stimulation will all encourage the release of the birthing hormones. Avoiding the Fight or Flight reflex by

keeping the BW free from disturbance, distraction or fear is possibly the best way to ensure these hormones pulse and flow in the way they need to.

7. Relax! What better time than the early phase of birth to practise hypnobirthing breathing and relaxation techniques. As your body warms up for birth you can take the time to get to that pleasant and comfortable place in your mind. See this as practice time though, it's not quite time yet but when it is you will be ready.

Chapter Twenty Four

The Active Phase of Birthing

As the surges open the neck of the womb wider they will take on a rhythm and become more regular. They will also become stronger and longer. In the majority of births there needs to be this regularity in the muscular action of the womb in order to pull the neck of the womb open so it becomes fully dilated. BW are very often aware of the changes in their body and the surges as their birthing becomes more active. They will sense that the surges are stronger and more frequent and may be aware of the baby moving lower by feeling pressure on the back passage or a heaviness or pressure on the perineum and in the vagina. Birthing partners might notice a change in the BW too. Maybe she says that things feel different and expresses that the surges are becoming more powerful. It might be that the BP notices the BW goes more 'within' and becomes more focused as she needs to pay more attention to the sensations. It could also be that she asks for more support and wants to use hypnobirthing techniques to stay focused and relaxed or that her breathing becomes much deeper particularly during a surge.

4 Top Tips for the Active Phase of birth

1. Drink! Dehydration in the BW will cause her to feel tired and ill. Around 55% of the adult female body is made up of water and in a newborn it can be as much as 80%! It is a vital energy source for the human body and during birth it is needed more than ever. If a BW becomes dehydrated her unborn baby's heart rate will rise and the baby will become tachycardic. It is also likely that the birthing will slow or even stop altogether as the body becomes low on the fuel it needs. To avoid all of this the BW should take on plenty of fluids. Water, ice, fruit juices, fruit smoothies and herbal

teas are all good. Crunching ice can be refreshing and can be helpful if there is any nausea.

Tip: Keep a sports or sippy bottle with you all the time and sip water between every surge

2. Eat! Take in easily digestible, high energy foods. Your body needs energy from calories to function well. Taking in fluid and calories will keep your energy levels up. The motility of the digestive system tends to slow down whilst birthing and this can mean the birthing woman's appetite can sometimes be reduced. It's important, though to take in calories in order to energise the body. Eating easily digestible, high energy foods regularly in small amounts usually works well.

Tip: For an easily digestible, energy power pack combine yoghurt, granola, honey and banana. For an energy boosting drink try the smoothie recipe below;

A handful of fresh pineapple, chopped
A handful of fresh watermelon, chopped
300mls of coconut water
A handful of baby spinach
A handful or frozen blueberries
2 bananas

Blend all the ingredients adding some crushed ice if desired.

3. Move! Moving for birth is discussed in detail in Chapter Twenty Two.

4. Breathe and relax. At a number of the hypnobirths I have attended I have been surprised at how little the couples used actual hypnobirthing techniques and yet still had amazing births. One such birth was the home birth/waterbirth/

hypnobirth of Amanda, where despite there being her birthing partner (Seth), two midwives and two other relatives present, there was total silence in the room for most of the time. From time to time Seth would make a round of tea and toast but otherwise we just sat and waited in comfortable silence. Although Seth didn't say much he stayed right by Amanda's side and was very much part of a shared experience. His focus was solely on Amanda and he appeared to observe her closely, I'm sure he would have responded immediately to any request she might have made. Earlier in the day before myself and my colleague arrived he had taken time to create a tranquil and cosy atmosphere in the room. He had lit a number of candles, dimmed the lights, gathered lots of cushions and blankets, made energising snacks, filled a hot water bottle and put on a track of birdsong on. The result was that the room felt relaxing and safe and a group of relative strangers could all be together in peace. Most importantly it meant that Amanda could feel safe and free of distractions, allowing her birthing body to get on with the job in hand without disruptions or interference.

Throughout the birth Amanda didn't want or ask for anything. Seth told me afterwards that they had practised breathing and relaxation techniques together nearly everyday for around two months in the run up to the birth. He also said that he was surprised that Amanda didn't ask to use these techniques or at least listen to the hypnobirthing CD that she had listened to everyday for the last eight weeks. It seems that for Amanda all the work had been done in that preparation, her mind was in the right place to be able to just relax and let it happen and nothing more was needed to be done.

This will not be the case with all hypnobirths of course. Some couples will find using the techniques during the birthing to be invaluable and necessary for calmness and positive thinking. One couple relating their hypnobirth story told how they played their hypnobirthing CD on a loop for the whole 9 hours of the birth, the hypnobirthing mum told me that as long as she could hear the words of the track she knew she could do it. Another couple described how they used a whole variety of techniques that they had learnt and practised and for them moving around the different techniques really worked. All these couples followed their instincts and did what felt right at the time. Whilst preparing for their hypnobirth couples should practise as many of the techniques as possible so they have them all at their disposal should they want them. If there are one or two techniques that really appeal and work well for the couple they may choose to focus on those and become really practised at them or they might prefer to have a wider variety of techniques to hand during the birth.

BW and their partners will often ask at what point the techniques should be used during the birth, the answer is whenever you feel like it! Birthing women are very instinctive and the subconscious will know what the BW needs and when to help her to relax deeply. There is no right or wrong, good or bad time to use the techniques, you can't start too early or leave it too late, you can't do too little or too much. Just as the BW will know when she is thirsty and needs to drink or needs to move to get more comfortable or needs the loo because she has a full bladder, so too she will know what she needs to be calm and confident.

When will we know it is time to call the midwife/go to hospital?

This is possibly one of the most commonly asked questions about managing the practicalities of a birthing. Birthing women and their partners are often keep to avoid calling the midwife too early to their home birth or arriving in hospital only to be sent home again. Women who are listening to their body and who are truly in touch with their birth will instinctively know when the time is right. The sensations of the surges and of the baby moving down will take their attention and require their focus and somehow they will just know. The reality is, though, when the BW speaks to her midwife to say she thinks her birthing is in the active phase the midwife is going to be very interested in the timing of the surges. A sensible, intelligent midwife will also take into account other signs such pressure on the back passage or a fullness in the vagina but ultimately he or she will want to know how often the surges are coming and how long they last. Midwives measure surges by how many occur in any ten minute time slot. So, for example, they may talk about surges being 3 in 10 which means there are 3 whole surges every 10 minutes. If you tell them the surges are 3 or 4 in 10 minutes and they are 1 minute long each and that it's been like that for a couple of hours with a first baby (about an hour with subsequent babies) they would say that it's likely that the active phase of birth has begun. This is important to know because it is almost inevitable that a conversation with you midwife will involve a discussion about time. However, as already mentioned earlier the principle of the BW dismissing time and letting her body tell her when it is time to birth does fly in the face of all this somewhat! To get round this dilemma I suggest the following.

1. The BW forgets about time, as the birthing begins she should remove her watch, turn round the clocks, switch off the TV and phones etc.

2. The BP stays close by the BW, listens to and observes her closely.

3. When the BW expresses that the surges have become powerful and regular or when she shows signs of the birth becoming more active (see page 148) or when the surges appear to be strong and rhythmical the BP should quietly and discreetly time the surges for just 20 minutes. There's no need to discuss the timing of each surge, this is potentially too distracting for the BW, instead the BP should calmly keep a mental note of how many surges there are and how long each one lasts.

4. If the surges are regular, that is, there are 3 or more every ten minutes and they each last a minute long the BP should wait half an hour to an hour and then once again quietly time the surges for another twenty minutes.

5. If the surges are not regular then the BP should wait until there are more signs of the active phase of birthing before timing again.

6. Once the regular surges have been going for an hour or two give the midwife a call and talk it through.

IMPORTANT NOTE: If any of the surges are accompanied by lots of pressure on the back passage and a strong urge to push, do not wait but call your midwife straight away. The likelihood is that the active phase of birth will take a few hours but occasionally it moves quicker. Lots of pressure and a feeling of bearing down may mean you are ready to birth.

FINAL NOTE: Many midwives will still use the level of a woman's pain and discomfort as one of the main parts of their assessment to ascertain whether or not she is in the active part of her birth. It is not unusual for midwives to be surprised at how far on in their birth or how dilated hypnobirthing women are as they do not appear to be distressed or in pain, in other words they just seem to be too comfortable. When the hypnobirthing couple speak to their midwife to say the birthing has become more active they should be clear first of all that they are using hypnobirthing and, therefore, might appear to be more comfortable than the midwife is used to. Secondly, let them know about the regularity and power of the surges, if you tell the midwife you have had powerful, long and regular surges for the last two hours it will make things clearer for him/ her. If by any chance your midwife has not heard of hypnobirthing tell her that you have been using specialized relaxation and hypnosis and breathing techniques for birth (and then give them this book to read!)

Afterword

Once a midwife colleague came to find me after witnessing her first hypnobirth. She was flushed with excitement as she described quite poetically, a peaceful, serene and gentle waterbirth. She had been a midwife for 25 years and said she had never seen anything like it before. 'You know', she said, 'it reminded me of why I became a midwife...I think I'd forgotten.'

The very next day I met a woman in our local park who had had her second baby using hypnobirthing just 6 days earlier. After I had admired the delightfully precious infant contentedly curled up in the sling we chatted for a while about her Home/ Hypno/Waterbirth. In just 4 hours she had birthed her son into the water without needing or wanting anything. As she finished and turned to leave she swung back for a moment and said, almost urgently, 'Judith, you've got to tell other women, there is another way!'

The Last Word

Remember this, all you have to do is breathe and let go, everything else will follow.

References

Albers L (2007) The Evidence for Physiologic Management of the Active Phase of the First Stage of Labor Journal of Midwifery & Women's Health 52: 207-215

Anderson, T (2002) “Out of the darkened room and into the laboratory” MIDIRS Midwifery Digest 12:1 pp. 65-69.

Bailit JL, Dierker L, Blanchard, Mercer B. (2005) Outcomes of women presenting in active versus latent phases of spontaneous labour. Obstetrics and Gynaecology 105(1): 77-79.

Baumgartner T, Heinr, Heinrichs M, Vonlanthen A, Fischbacher U, Fehr E. (2008), Oxytocin Shapes the Neural Circuitry of Trust and TrustAdaptation in Humans, Neuron 58(4), 639-650.

Carmichael MS, Humbert R, Dixen J, Palmisano G, Greenleaf W, Davidson JM (January 1987). "Plasma oxytocin increases in the human sexual response". The Journal of Clinical Endocrinology and Metabolism 64 (1): 27–31.

Cea Ugarte JI., Gonzalez-Pinto Arrillaga A., Cabo Gonzalez OM. (2010) Efficacy of the controlled breathing therapy on stress: biological correlates. Escuela de Enfermería. Revista de Enfermería;33(5):48-54.

Chang, M.Y., Wang, S. Y., & Chen, C. H. (2002). Effects of massage on pain and anxiety during labour: a randomised controlled trial in Taiwan. Journal of Advanced Nursing 38 (1), 68-73.

Chang, Mei-Yueh, Chung-Hey Chen, Kuo-Feng Huang. (2006) “A comparison of massage effects on labor pain using the Mcgill Pain questionnaire." Journal of Nursing Research vol. 14, No.3.

Cluett, E. R.; Burns, E. (2009). Immersion in water in labour and birth. In Cluett, Elizabeth R. "Cochrane Database of Systematic Reviews". Cochrane database of systematic reviews (Online) (2)

Contos K, Rust M, Höllt V. (1981) The role of endorphins during parturition.NIDA Res Monogr. Feb;34:264-71.

Dick-Read, Grantly (2004), (Eds) Childbirth without Fear: The Principles and Practice of Natural Childbirth,. Pinter & Martin.

Ditzen B, et al (2008), Intranasal Oxytocin Increases Positive Communication and Reduces Cortisol Levels During Couple Conflict. Biological Psychiatry, 65(9): 728–731.

Downe S (Ed), (2004) Normal Childbirth: Evidence and Debate, Churchill Livinstone. Chapter 2, The role of pain in normal birth and the empowerment of women, Leap N, Anderson, T.

Durand, Mark A. (1992). The Safety of Home Birth: The Farm Study, American Journal of Public Health, 82:450-452.

Foster, Dr.; Smith, Dr.. "Purring in Cats".
www.peteducation.com/article.cfm? Retrieved 2011-04-10.
Accessed 2012

Gaskin IM (2008) (Eds) Ina May's Guide to Childbirth,, Vermillion.

Gaskin IM (2002). (Eds) Spiritual midwifery, 4th edition. USA: Book Publishing Company.

Holmes P, Oppenheimer L, Wen S (2001) The relationship between cervical dilatation at initial presentation in labour and subsequent intervention British Journal of Obstetrics and Gynaecology 108: 1120-1124.

Horace H. Loh, L. F. Tseng, Eddie Wei, and Choh Hao Li (1976). Beta-endorphin is a potent analgesic agent. PNAS 73 (8): 2895–2898.

Kaushik, R.M., Kaushik, R., Mahajan, S.K., et al. (2006). Effects of mental relaxation and slow breathing in essential hypertension. Complimentary Therapies in Medicine. Jun; 14(2):120-6.

Klein M, Kelly A, Koczorowski J, Grzybowski S (2004) The effect of camily physician timing of maternal admission on procedures in labour and maternal and infant morbidity. Journal of Obstetrics and Gynaecology Canada 26(7): 641-645.

Martin, C. (2009), Effects of Valsalva manoeuvre on maternal and fetal wellbeing, British Journal of Midwifery, vol. 17, no. 5, pp. 279-85.

Meyer, Dixie (2007). "Selective Serotonin Reuptake Inhibitors and Their Effects on Relationship Satisfaction". The Family Journal 15 (4): 392–397.

NCCWCH. (2007). Intrapartum care: care of healthy women and their babies during childbirth. National Collaborating Centre for Women's and Children's Health. Clinical Guidelines. London: RCOG Press.

Nolan M, Smith J. (2010) Women's experiences of following advice to stay at home in early labour. British Journal of Midwifery; 18(5):286-91.

O'Donnell K, O'Connor T. G, Glover V (2009). Prenatal stress and neurodevelopment of the child: focus on the HPA axis and role of the placenta. Dev Neurosci. 31(4):285-92.

Rahm V, (2002) Plasma oxytocin levels in women during labor with or without epidural analgesia: a prospective study. Acta Obstetricia et Gynecologica Scandinavica 81(11):1033–1039.

Robertson, D. (2009) The Complete Writings of James Braid the Father of Hypnotherapy National Council for Hypnotherapy Ltd.; 1st edition

Rosenthal, R. (2003). Covert communication in laboratories, classrooms, and the truly real world. Psychological Science, 12, 151-155

Scaglione R, Cummins W, (1993) Karate of Okinawa: Building Warrior Spirit, Tuttle Publishing.

Sharkey J T, Puttaramu, R. Word, R. Olcese J (2009) Melatonin Synergizes with Oxytocin to Enhance Contractility of Human Myometrial Smooth Muscle Cells. J Clin Endocrinol Metab. 94(2): 421–427.

Simkin, P., and Bolding, A., (2004). Update on Non-pharmacologic Approaches to Relieve Labor Pain and Prevent Suffering. Journal of Midwifery and Womens" Health. Nov/Dec. 49 (6), 496.

Spinelli A, Bagli G, Grandolfo ME and Osborn J, (2003) "Do antenatal classes benefit mother and her baby?" Journal of Maternal and Neonatal Medicine Feb: 13(2): 94-101.

Van der Donck A, "A Description of the New Netherlands," 2d ed. (Amsterdam, 1656), trans. Jeremiah Johnson, in Collections of the New-York Historical Society, 2d series, 1 (1841).

WHO (1996) Care in Normal Birth: a Practice Guide.

http://www.guardian.co.uk/lifeandstyle/2009/sep/26/natural-birth-expert

http://www.unicef.org.uk/BabyFriendly/Resources/Guidance-for-Health-Professionals/Learning-about-breastfeeding/Skin-to-skin-contact/

Judge's order in full.
http://ttabvue.uspto.gov/ttabvue/v?pno=92032066&pty=CAN&eno=19

http://www.rcmnormalbirth.org.uk/

http://www.rcmnormalbirth.org.uk/stories/if-at-first/second-stage-pushing/

http://www.homebirth.org.uk/ofp.htm

http://www.clinical-depression.co.uk/dlp/depression-information/medical-causes-of-depression/ Accessed 2012